The Role of Trust in Mental Health

This book offers a comprehensive examination of trust and its relationship with mental illness and wellbeing.

Engaging with a broad range of mental health research, theory, and practice through various transdisciplinary theoretical models of trust, this book highlights the social and family contexts surrounding the making and breaking of trust and mental health. It examines various sociological conceptual and theoretical frameworks of risk and trust while also engaging with evolutionary perspectives on the human need for cooperation and trust. The author describes how, in a world of constant connectivity, the drawing of boundaries assigns some people as strangers, using stigma as a form of power. The book concludes by considering the future of mental health and where trust-building may be possible. Each chapter is interspersed with observations and insights from the author's personal research covering many populations, communities, and issues over several decades.

Drawing on a wide range of interdisciplinary literature, the book will be of interest to mental health practitioners, researchers, and scholars interested in the psychosocial aspects of mental illness and stigma.

Gerard Leavey has researched and published widely on mental illness and health inequalities. His work spans health service and epidemiological studies on ethnicity, suicide, and severe mental illness and qualitative investigations of religious leaders, and schoolteachers, and their role in the recognition and management of mental illness. His current work is focussed on tackling the social exclusion of people with severe mental illness.

'Professor Leavey's book throws light on a far too long neglected factor with a powerful impact on structures of society and the management of problems ranging from care for people with diseases to the continuation of war or the maintenance of peace'.

– **Professor Norman Sartorius** (MD, PhD, FRCPsych) is a leading international expert in psychiatry. He has been the President of the World Psychiatric Association and of the European Psychiatric Association, and Director of the Mental health Division of the World Health Organization.

'Trust is one of those concepts that we make assumptions about throughout our academic writing. As so eloquently told in this book, we often forget the role of trust in building health and wellbeing, or conversely, how mistrust is so corrosive to social bonds and healthy minds. Professor Leavey's book on trust and mental illness is written with considerable skill and knowledge on a wide range of subjects and issues. It provides an excellent reflection on the source of many of our social and psychological problems but also offers sound advice on how to mitigate them'.

– **Seeromanie Harding** is Professor of Social Epidemiology at King's College London, where she leads the Population Health and Nutrition Research group. Her expertise spans social and ethnic inequalities in health over the life course, international comparative studies, and community-based interventions in low-resource settings. Her research covers complex socio-cultural-political contexts that drive health disparities.

'In this book, Professor Gerard Leavey describes, probes, unpicks and reveals to the reader the crucial place that trust occupies in relation to mental health and mental illness. Going way beyond the basic concept of 'therapeutic alliance' that the title might imply, he addresses the concept at multiple levels (individual, interpersonal, societal, political, philosophical...) and engages the reader in a heady and immersive contextualisation of why trust matters. For anyone interested in learning more about the impact of the social world on mental health, add this to your reading list!'

– **Professor Helen Killaspy** is a clinical academic working in the field of rehabilitation psychiatry. Her research has provided crucial evidence for the effectiveness of specialist services for people with complex mental health needs. She has played a key role in ensuring this evidence is included in policy to support ongoing investment in mental health rehabilitation services internationally. In 2019, the European Psychiatric Association awarded her the Constance Pascal-Helen Boyle Prize for Outstanding Achievement by a Woman in Working to Improve Mental Health Care in Europe. In 2021, she received a Lifetime Achievement Award from the Faculty of Rehabilitation and Social Psychiatry of the UK Royal College of Psychiatrists.

'This remarkable book takes the concepts of trust and mental health and moves them around each other as if they were reciprocal moons of our planetary existence. Trust is a concept perfectly central to individuals, families, communities and society. For almost a thousand years the idea of 'trust' has grown from the ancient roots of meaning that include: integrity, alliance, faithful, steadfast, shelter, safety, hope, and consolation. This book is a fascinating tour-de-force which gazes at trust and hope, and their inversions, from multiple perspectives, and asks how we can strengthen trust and hope and mental health in the future'.

– **Sir Graham Thornicroft** is Emeritus Professor of Community Psychiatry at King's College London. He was Knighted in 2017 for services to mental health; Graham has authored over 30 books and written over 670 peer-reviewed scientific papers, shaping global mental health policies.

The Role of Trust in Mental Health

Vulnerability and Trust-Building in Theory and Practice

Gerard Leavey

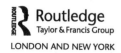 Routledge
Taylor & Francis Group

LONDON AND NEW YORK

Cover image: Albrecht Dürer: Melencolia I

First published 2025
by Routledge
4 Park Square, Milton Park, Abingdon, Oxon OX14 4RN

and by Routledge
605 Third Avenue, New York, NY 10158

Routledge is an imprint of the Taylor & Francis Group, an informa business

British Library Cataloguing-in-Publication Data
A catalogue record for this book is available from the British Library

ISBN: 978-1-032-35394-4 (hbk)
ISBN: 978-1-032-35387-6 (pbk)
ISBN: 978-1-003-32668-7 (ebk)

DOI: 10.4324/9781003326687

Typeset in Times New Roman
by KnowledgeWorks Global Ltd.

Contents

Preface

Over three decades my research in mental health and health services covered a considerable range of people and diagnoses, populations and communities, beliefs, and behaviours. From the miseries and uncertainties of adolescents to the miseries and uncertainties of old age and dementia, I have been intrigued by the challenges of each and how best to ameliorate them. The pace of academic life, speeding from one research grant and publication to another, often stultifies the creative imagination, blinding one to the many other possible threads that connect disparate populations and disorders. After all, what are the shared factors between the poor social and health outcomes of young black men, and the reluctance of adolescents to contact their family doctors? Or what is the connection between the depression and suicide of Irish migrant workers in London and their upbringing in Ireland? Why do so many good teachers find their work stressful and quit the profession? Only retrospectively did I consider the underlying influence of trust and mistrust in determining mental illness and what to do about it.

The dismal explanation for its absence is that trust is seldom measured in mental health research. If trust isn't measured, then it is likely that it isn't considered salient, or alternatively perhaps, it may be regarded as too complex or slippery to capture. I suggest that trust may be a concept that is so embedded in everyday discourse but with so little clarity that its taken-for-granted quality escapes any real scrutiny in healthcare research, relative to its significance within political or business studies. Research that fully appreciates the importance of trust in mental illness, the provision of mental health services and the development of trust-informed interventions, remain underdeveloped. The reasons for this perhaps lie in the scattering of the concept across disciplines, its implicit value in other concepts, and the significant overshadowing of trust that this produces.

The disjunction between qualitative and quantitative research and the mutual contempt commonly held by researchers from these camps is partly to blame. In qualitative research, especially where the focus is on the individual, the data collected pertain to the subjective accounts of participants who have been asked to describe and explain their values, beliefs, attitudes, and experiences about phenomena, or in relation to their life stories. As an inductive methodology, the researcher approaches the interviewee without any predetermined questions but rather with an open curiosity which allows the interviewee (or participant) to reveal what is of importance and to explain why. Of course, subjective revelations tend not to be uncontrolled verbal outpourings of participants, but rather, are usually guided through light but semi-structured open-ended questioning by sensitive and thoughtful researchers, hopefully. Out of rivers of text, the researcher seeks to identify precious explanatory nuggets, the themes that illuminate our understanding of the phenomena in question and the factors that relate to them. If done well, by which I mean with substantial depth and richness, qualitative research should provide a deepening of theory. However, despite the vital knowledge contribution of qualitative research, it is still prone to bias in various forms including confirmation bias – the researcher 'finds' what he/she is interested in and filters out, consciously or unconsciously, those data that don't fit. In other instances, the researcher may simply miss the connective tissue or threads that appear in different participant accounts or misperceive a distal or underlying construct.

The growing pressure for rapid and brief publications creates the ingredients for an under-engagement with complex issues. In my own case, the salience of loneliness or trust in the lives of people with mental illness was emulsified in the overall description but never the central feature made invisible in the process. Quantitative research is bedevilled by similar problems. While trust in institutions, clinicians, and services is a major factor in how people seek help, access, and engage with services, or respond to clinical advice and treatment, measures of trust are inadequately developed and seldom considered for use. Trust as a construct is often assumed to be present in measures of satisfaction with psychiatric services or mistakenly substituted with confidence in the clinician. It isn't.

I hope that future health service researchers will bring trust into the conceptualisation of their work, rather than as an afterthought in the write-up.

Acknowledgements

Thanks to Hannah and my children Cara, Nina, Esther and Reuben – always interested, patient, and supportive.

I would like to dedicate this book in memory of
Professor Michael King (University College London),
who gave me much and so generously.

Chapter 1

Introduction

Trust in our major social institutions is widely described to be in crisis – variously threatened by social change, globalism, and digital technology, not to mention institutional self-harm. The nature and mechanisms of trust itself has been transformed by our relationship with increasingly complex and abstract systems (Giddens, 1991). The modern individual is enveloped includes the ever-burgeoning World Wide Web and the dizzying growth of the internet dominated by globally powerful and all-pervasive multinational digital-based corporations. Modernity also means that we are connected to distant networks of political, economic, and cultural forces, which appear difficult to locate and harder to control.

Moreover, the growth of the internet and digital technology provokes anxiety about their potential to fast-track the realisation of post-modernist ideas, facilitating human retreat into a near solipsistic and virtual universe in which 'truths' are eclectic and a la carte and where science may simply be discarded as one narrative among many; no single overarching truth and no way to sift out the nuggets from the dross. Perhaps most remarkably, these and other forces summon the potential emergence of the truly private individual whose affective, economic, intellectual, and material needs find satisfaction entirely at home, intersecting with the interests of other like-minded individuals, who are equally devoid of demands and commitments. A flow of ideas and concepts, interests, connections, and stories can be engaged momentarily or stitched together by detached individuals. Lyotard (1994) suggests a world stripped of a *grand narrative*, where a myriad of non-superior narratives jostle for attention, the individual has nowhere to go other than a place of his or her choosing. In just over a hundred years, all kinds of seemingly invincible monolithic institutions have faded away or completely collapsed overnight. In the 21st century, polls consistently and reliably show a withering of trust in politicians and political institutions in the United States and elsewhere.[1] Free markets, industrial automation, and social inequalities are thought to further deplete popular trust in its politicians and institutions and the polarisation of citizens.

The penetration of such forces into everyday existence has implications for the mental health of individuals and communities but may deplete the wellbeing of social trust. If our anxiety is commensurate with the perceived threat from others, the more likely our withdrawal and retreat behind increasing defensive structures,

DOI: 10.4324/9781003326687-1

producing more isolation and loss of social cooperation. Everything that we know or intuit about the protection of mental health tells us that this is not salutogenic.

Trust and mental health

Until recently, trust was relatively absent in the sociological literature, a 'silent presence' as Misztal described it, only detected in key sociological writings analysing the transition from pre-modern to modern society (Giddens, 1991). Although extensive academic and public discussion is focussed on institutional trust, predominantly related to concerns about citizens' engagement with social, political, and economic activities, only recently has interdisciplinary interest surfaced on trust in healthcare. Perhaps surprisingly, much less attention has been paid to the role of trust in the development and management of mental health, wellbeing, and illness. Surprising for many reasons, but not least because trust and mental health intersect deeply at key political and philosophical questions about the nature of reality, equality, freedom, responsibility, beliefs, and punishment among other things. Similar to Misztal's observation, the varied, often disguised, appearance of trust (and mistrust possibly more so) is detectable through its traces in the development and treatment of mental illnesses and the lives of those affected by them – which means most of us. Saturating almost every dimension of human existence from birth to death, every outcome considered important to most people, from basic needs to health and life satisfaction, is influenced by the presence or absence of trust.[2]

The costs of the illness to individuals and families can be immense, all-consuming, and long-lasting. For society, mental disorders worldwide account for 32% of years of disability and 13% of disability adjusted life years (Vigo et al., 2016). Moreover, despite much vaunted public policies on improving the wellbeing of citizens, evidence suggests that most of us are increasingly depressed, anxious, and stressed, and particularly pervasive in the lives of young people. Loneliness too, we are informed, has reached epidemic proportions, as prevalent among adolescents if not more so than among the elderly. There exists an extensive range of psychiatric disorders, many of them common – the symptoms of which are experienced by most of us at some level, while others are rare but more consequential in how they impact the lives of individuals and their families. In both the more commonly experienced and rare forms of mental health problems, the fragility or absence of trust overshadows the development of the illness, its course, management, and outcomes. In different illnesses, the experience and meaning of trust-mistrust in the lives of patients are both causal and consequential, a failure to trust or the destruction of trust engendered by the actions or inactions of others, leaving the individual lonely and alienated.

In the lives of people devoid of trust or simply denied the ability and inclination to develop trust, the capacity for meaningful, mature, and positive relationships is stunted. For other people, suspicion and mistrust, paranoid thoughts and feelings are central to their illness experiences. Of course, there may be something in the individual's history, a traumatic event predisposing them to mistrust, and provoking lifelong hypervigilance to external harms, but it is the extreme and delusional dimensions of mistrust in the expression of paranoia, so characteristic of schizophrenia, that are usually considered in the literature, largely differentiated from neurotic symptoms and behaviours. While noting this categorical boundary, it is also true that while there are major qualitative differences in the expression and outcomes of neurotic and psychotic disorders, there is also evidence that there may be considerable overlap in their causal events and circumstances and that mistrustfulness is common to both.

Whenever trust is discussed in the context of mental illness, as in other areas of healthcare, it usually pertains to patients' assessment of clinicians and treatment. With some exceptions, the examination of trust and mental illness tends to get stranded somewhat in research on professions and the institution (Pilgrim et al., 2011). Also neglected is how the conditions for trust and the creation of (mis)trusting individuals may be established from birth, perhaps much earlier. Missing too is the role of trust (and mistrust) in determining health inequalities across diverse social groups, whether based on social class or ethnicity, or both. The higher rates of schizophrenia among some ethnic communities compared to their white counterparts and low rates of help-seeking suggest a problematic trust relationship with mental health services.

The stranger

Explored by the social thinker George Simmel,[3] the stranger is defined by distance – he or she can never occupy a position which is too close or too far, in that with proximity and intimacy comes knowledge and connection and thus membership of the group. Too distant from the group, the individual has no contact and is erased from consciousness. However, the relationship of the stranger to the group allows certain privileged perspectives on its actions. Thus, sitting outside the group, the stranger may have greater objectivity than any particular individual within the group – that is, in acknowledging the stranger's neutrality to the group's relationships, the stranger can be relied upon to provide disinterested advice, rather in the same way that one might speak to a psychotherapist who similarly occupies a transitional space, or attempts to guide the individual through a transitional state. However, the stranger in many societies continues to provoke not just interest but varying levels of mistrust and hostility at interpersonal, social, and political levels.

Modern Western liberal societies since the late 20th century have been characterised by increasing diversity of identity in its myriad forms – gender, sexuality, ethnic, and religion – with varying degrees of successful and harmonious acceptance. Unfortunately, the demand for social, sometimes legal, recognition continues to provoke a backlash from various sectors who regard the assertion for recognition and rights as a moral threat to traditional values and norms. Charles Taylor in his discussion of contemporary politics and the demand by identity-based groups for recognition argues that in the premodern age, 'identity' and 'recognition' were not discussion topics 'not because people didn't have (what we call) identities, or because these didn't depend on recognition, but rather because these were then too unproblematic to be thematized as such' (Taylor, 2021). Thus, the social categories that people assumed, existed simply because they were taken for granted. By and large, people were defined by their family and their occupation; they may have been liked or disliked, trusted or not, but did not struggle with issues of individual identity. In any case identity, bound as it was to family and place, left little room for betrayal of trust produced collective consequences.

The modern ideal of authenticity, self-realisation, and self-fulfilment, Taylor argues, requires of the individual a truthfulness to oneself which only they can articulate and in doing so, become self-defining. The multifarious choices and opportunities created by modernity create a palette from which to draw a self-definition, which may not be static either. While Taylor recognises the importance of equal recognition in a 'healthy democratic society', the refusal of which 'can inflict damage on those who are denied it' and that the 'withholding of recognition can be a form of oppression' (Taylor, 2021, p. 31). What constitutes a 'health democratic society' is debatable, but by most reasonable definitions, this appears currently fragile in most Western nation states. Moreover, matters of identity and belonging have been co-opted into the polarising politics of the age. The importance of the concepts of identity and diversity concern issues of equity and justice, and the challenges for developing trust at social, institutional, and personal levels. The conflicts that arise from issues of identity are precisely epitomised by the rapid appearance and politically contested nature of gender identity.

Throughout this book, I suggest that trust and mistrust are central to the development of mental illness and the lifeworld of people who must live with these conditions. My aim is to explore how various psychiatric disorders, symptoms, and manifestations are shaped, determined, and often reflected by social and psychological dimensions of trust. Although perhaps impossible to determine the optimal environment and circumstances from which a 'healthy' trust emerges, we have reasonable evidence about the factors that stunt or erode trust formation necessary for social and personal wellbeing. While trust may be important to social engagement and exchange, trust can sometimes be misplaced and dangerous. Certainly, there are bad actors, treacherous environments, and unknown factors which elevate the possibility of risk, rendering trust as a foolish bet. Environments, including home and home life that foster a healthy trust are those that prepare the individual for useful, productive, and moral engagement with society, mitigating exposure to an omnipresent or inappropriate anxieties. In this sense, trust, or at least, the calculation of trust, is accommodated by culture as a 'toolkit' (Swidler, 1986), a set of skills and knowledge that permits useful participation in any society and Pierre Bourdieu's *habitus* (Bourdieu, 1977) – dispositions to the relational structures through which the individual is both socialised in a given society and reshapes it.

Without trust, the world-building task of the individual in society would be even more challenging than it is or might never get started. A useful approach to understanding the relationship between individual actors and the external world, habitus acknowledges the exchange between material and subjective realities. Acting in the world with trust is largely done unconsciously, behaving with an internalised knowledge that requires no premeditation; if it were otherwise much of our actions, even the mundane ones would grind to paralysis. Moreover, much of what we have learned in childhood about the environment is felt, experienced bodily rather than taught. We react to unusual smells – especially heightened when they suggest something dangerous, something rotten – literally and metaphorically, we 'smell a rat'. As Camus suggests in The Myth of Sisyphus (Camus, 2005), 'The body's judgement is as good as the mind's and the body shrinks from annihilation. We get into the habit of living before we get into the habit of thinking'. However, in a complex world of increasing threats and related anxieties such as those posed by conflict, pandemics, or climate-related ecological catastrophes, the propensity to mistrust, to shrink from annihilation, imposes upon the individual an anomic world of loneliness with an accompanying loss of self and meaning. However, engagement with society also means that our knowledge of and responses to our worlds are contextual and contingent, requiring adjustment in the light of new knowledge of other factors and change. Thus, the individual's navigation of the social world, although unconscious, is tested continually, absorbing and recalibrating.

In some respects, this book is an attempt to understand the issue of trust and mental health from the 'elsewhere' which I consider to be the social determinants located in social adversity. The development of mental illness can only be understood as the interface between our genes and the environment, nature and nurture. Accepting that all human beings, to different degrees, have an inherited vulnerability to this or that mental illness, exposure to events, behaviours, and circumstances may tip the scales towards actual pathology. Individual characteristics may divert some people entirely from a mental illness, or mitigate the damage done, providing resilience for others. Throughout various chapters and using examples from research, the concept of trust is explored within these exposures and how individuals and social groups are impacted by them. In doing so, I suggest that we must consider trust as a relational concept in which the consideration of the psychology of individuals, their cognitions, emotions, and behaviours is appropriately done through a social lens. While the tendency to trust or mistrust is not completely determined by our genetic inheritance, it is obvious that as social animals our evolution has benefited from the 'instinct' to cooperate with some people but judiciously avoid others as much as possible. A shorthand solution to dealing with the risk posed by others in situations of vulnerability is to gravitate trustingly towards others who appear similar to us, avoiding the unknowability of multiple others. The gravitation towards some people and the avoidance of others may also be misguided. Thus, while trust-building between social actors serves the purpose of obtaining cooperation towards a desired outcome, the motivation of those wishing to be trusted, their motivation in doing so may not be authentically benign, they may simply be astute in faking trustworthiness.

Even though the heritability of mental illness lurks in the background for most people, the development of a psychiatric disorder remains contingent, not least upon the social and relationship dimensions of human development, particularly love and respect within a trusting and secure environment. At the wider macro-level, it is difficult to see how human organisation and flourishing is possible in the absence of a 'secure base', to use John Bowlby's phrase (1988). Our ontological security needs a home, a place from which we set out and return, if we are fortunate. What if the homes or communities in which we are raised are not oriented to the development of confident, resilient, integrated, and contented individuals? What is the impact of disadvantage and adversity on one's perceptions of the world and how to behave within it? Indeed, as explored in this book, violence and conflict, as a rupture, not only in the normal circumstances of upbringing but also within community and national contexts, can have detrimental impacts, either experienced as unexpected and abrupt departures from the norm or as slowly observed and corrosive, on both one's trust in the world and one's mental health. Again, throughout various chapters, I use a historical and life-course perspective that suggests that wellbeing and trust (and mistrust) are not solely interpersonal, conveyed from one person to another, unaffected by identity, culture, history, or life events, but rather are processed by some or all of these in combination. In short, we find among different groups and communities, legacies of trust or mistrust, depending on these histories.

Giddens theoretical perspectives on modernity and trust – e.g. ontological security, self-identity, and abstract systems will be helpful in exploring the differences and connections between the aetiologies of mental disorders and the social and institutional responses to 'breakdown'. The historical perspective will, briefly, take the reader from a preindustrial, collective basis of trust, through to modern and post-modern discussion of the individual, self, and the fluid world of digital communication and the destabilisation of trust. I then outline the crucial and universal importance of trust for community, mental health and wellbeing, and the future of health services. Thus, trust is also central to matters of healthy social relations and upon whom or what we rely on for support in its different forms.

In Chapter 2, I explore the social dimensions of trust and the plausibility of *generalised trust*. Can members of any nation or community for that matter be said to have a measurable quotient of trust in their fellow citizens, or are we much more circumspect about whom we can trust, when and in what circumstances? Social cohesion, order, and authority are all predicated, to some degree, on trust. It is in this space that we touch upon arguably the most central of all sociological preoccupations – the maintenance of order. The behaviour of humans even in highly totalitarian societies is not programmable but nevertheless tends to be guided and shaped by innumerable micro-laws, generalised environmental expectations of how things are, and what will happen given this or that action. The routinization of life is usually determined within a particular set of cultural norms – polite behaviour in restaurants, orderly queuing at bus stops, or that our neighbours can be expected to not park their car in our driveway or invade our homes. Sometimes these expectations are underwritten by legislation – driving on the wrong side of the road or beating up one's children (or someone else's) tends to be frowned upon in most societies to varying degrees. International legislation and courts have been established in the hope of maintaining order or punishing transgression. Nevertheless, our implicit faith in that we will experience no harm or suffer a negative consequence in the undertaking of daily activities permits the free continuance of interactions with the environment and relationships. However, we can only discuss this level of trust in generalities; a desired state produced within ideal conditions. People and nations behave badly, traffic lights break down. Other actions that develop and bolster trust between individuals and their environment break down too, or never existed.

More positively, the notion of a generalised trust as a social good is firmly embedded in the concept of social capital derived from Bourdieu but made popular by Putnam – a kind of latent variable that links into and enhances the health, security, and prosperity of the community. Intuitively, this makes sense but as discussed in later chapters, social capital as an explanation for health inequalities is only partial, often obscuring the seminal cause of poverty. Throughout this book, many of the theoretical issues and themes related to trust are considered.

In Chapter 8, I argue that the origins of minority ethnic mistrust in psychiatry have been determined by complex historical forces that remain potent in their potential to contaminate relationships. While scientific racism was employed by colonialist powers for the denigration and mistrust of 'the other' as justification for the exploitation of colonised populations, the dynamics of mistrust continue to play out through intergenerational trauma and the highly conflicted relationship between minority ethnic groups and psychiatry – illustrated using examples from the United Kingdom and international literature. For example, many African Caribbean migrants who came to the United Kingdom in the 20th century – viewed England as the 'mother country', embodied for many decades by the Queen. The reality of their experiences of rejection and hostility has striking parallels with abusive parenting and the development of insecure attachment described by Bowlby and Winnicott. Other minority ethnic and religious communities distrust psychiatry due to differences in cultural beliefs and explanatory models of illness. In some faith-based communities, mistrust is often due to concerns for perceived anti-religious beliefs in psychiatry. In Chapter 8, I consider the breakdown of community's trust in the 'system', manifested in high rates of mental illness, incarceration, and fear of psychiatry.

Aliens and Alienists, the title of a book by academic psychiatrists Roland Littlewood and Maurice Lipsedge (1989), the former a renowned medical anthropologist, reminded us that an *alien* is an archaic term for a mentally ill person and an *alienist*, the term for a psychiatrist, particularly one who specialises in legally determining sanity and/or the capacity to stand trial for criminal offences. Although used as a critique of Western psychiatry's involvement in scientific racism and its legacy in current mental healthcare system, the use of the term *alien* encourages an exploration of the social and phenomenological experiences of alienation, the determinants of alienation and its impact on the individual and the community. However, the status of alien encompasses not just the marginalised individual with mental health problems but those whose problems are provoked by the processes of alienation within a given community or those people deemed to be alien by communities due to their national, ethnic, or cultural status.

Conflict, of which interpersonal and intercommunal violence are the most obvious and externalised dimensions, is a major determinant of mental illness. In psychoanalytic terms, conflict represents the pain of a new dynamic that emerges when two opposing energies collide. Thus, a patient's bodily complaints located in a particular organ may be the result of unconscious and/or undesirable desires and thoughts. Psychoanalysis point to the relevance of conflict in various areas of mental illness such as the presence of aggression redirected towards the self in depression and suicidality or converted into migraines (Bateman et al., 2000). As discussed in Chapter 4, much of the debilitating mental health problems experienced by many of us emerge out of our childhood relationships and which continue to influence the management of future relations and the negotiation of trust throughout life.

In Chapter 3, I examine interpersonal and social aspects in the relationship between trust and conflict. Jan Phillip Reemtsma (2012) in his introduction to *Trust and Violence* writes about continual human incredulity about human propensity for horrendous violence as though it comes as a renewed surprise to each generation, forgetting all previous acts of rage and brutality. Reetsma suggests that the focus of his interest is on the human capacity for a persistent trust in modernity despite our knowledge that conflict is the routine and natural state of the human condition rather than the unanticipated event it always seems to be. Like Vladimir and Estragon in Beckett's tragicomedy *Waiting for Godot* (Beckett, 2006), despite the lack of evidence that things will indeed get better, humans carry on. Reemtsma also argues that the separation out of trust into that which obtains at the institutional and the individual levels that there must be connective tissue between these. It makes no sense to 'speak of social trust if we didn't assume that it affected our behavioural expectations of others' (Reemtsma, 2012, p. 13). However, while acts of betrayal are often long remembered by individuals, commensurate with the original depth of relationship, the remembering of human propensity for violence is easily 'dis-owned' and dismissed as an aberration, a characteristic of others. I make the case that not only does violence and trauma shatter the individual's self-trust by destroying their assumptive worlds but also shatters the ambient social trust that may help recovery. While individual treatments such as post-traumatic stress disorder (PTSD) may be effective in attenuating individual symptoms they may also, inadvertently, create a market in 'victim-status' rather than resiliency-building and the pursuit of normalisation. Using Galtung's definitions of violence and peace, community-wide, justice-based approaches to trust-building may be more effective than reliance on individual treatments only. Thus, social capital approaches that focus on collective, holistic, and innovative programmes in which optimism, resilience, and new competencies are emphasised and likely to achieve much more in terms of interpersonal and generalised trust, personal and public security, growth, and health. I argue that a focus on individualised trauma gives a preferential position to individual treatment and may permit the channelling of resources away from more systemic healing modalities.

In Chapter 4, I explore the impacts of childhood adversity and mistrust across the life course. The work of Bowlby and others highlighted the connections between early childhood experiences and the individual's ability to explore and form healthy lasting relationships; the capacity to trust and to love oneself and others. In doing so, we are protected against lifetime problems of chronic loneliness and a range of health problems that are associated with isolation. People who have experienced childhood adversity also tend to mistrust other people, a behaviour which tends to result in loneliness, often across the life course. The conditions for trust and the creation of trusting individuals may be established from birth, perhaps even earlier, and in this, questions about the hard-wired or mutable nature of trust. Adverse childhood experiences and circumstances may profoundly influence a person's comprehension of, and attitudes to, the world, generalising from one's personal challenging experiences within family and immediate community to society generally with the expectation of similar treatment. The types of adverse events include witnessing parental marital discord and domestic violence, growing up with family members who have a mental illness or who have spent time in jail. Commonly, such events occur in clusters, and there is a dose-response relationship with increasingly negative health and social outcomes associated with multiple adversities (Curran et al., 2020).

Paradoxical, at first sight, perhaps there is some evidence that lonely adolescents report more 'friends' on the internet. It may be that the stigma attached to a perceived small friendship network is unbearable for many adolescents and too risky to expose. At the other end of the life spectrum are growing numbers of lonely older people who feel disconnected and threatened by technology. While there has been a major increase in the prevalence of mental illness among young people, especially adolescent girls, few will seek professional help.

In Chapter 5, drawing on my own research in this area, I explore the threats perceived by young people and their hypervigilant responses – what as Kleinman asks is 'at stake'? However, risk and trust in healthcare is double-edged. Not all patients are trusted as having valid medical or psychiatric issues. I explore the challenges faced by young people with gender identity dysphoria as they try to obtain medical and psychiatric intervention. Gender dysphoria is complex and highly contested – requiring professionals' acceptance and trust in the person's authenticity. Again, drawing on research in this area (including my own), I examine the patient-physician relationship and issues where risk and trust are problematic.

Trust is commonly reported as the cornerstone of medical relationships but has received scant attention in health research. Despite its importance in help-seeking, communication, decision-making, and patient engagement, trust is seldom measured as a determinant of health outcomes. In Chapter 6, I examine theory and determinants of healthcare trust and some of the threats to trust that arise from concerns about medical hegemony – the medicalisation of life problems – and how healthcare systems manage growing pluralism, misconduct, and conspiracy theories. If some form of 'thick trust' between people and institutions is predicated on 'familiarity', then the organisation of modern healthcare systems and increasing reliance on remote patient engagement may deplete patient-doctor trust.

Reality and madness

The words 'truth' and 'trust' have the same etymological roots in proto-Indo-European languages, traced to *deru* for tree – embracing meanings of solidity, reliability, and faithfulness. When family, community, and psychiatric professionals agree that an individual's behaviour can be deemed as an illness – stepping beyond the usual boundaries of what is expected from a member of that society and can agree what the most appropriate treatment should be, then there is potential for the development of trust between these different actors, even if the patient's interpretation and treatment is different. Problematically for society and those designated with managing the madness of citizens, the beliefs and behaviours of many citizens often fall within the considered boundaries of madness.

In various sections of this book, I explore the common-sense knowledge that constitutes the reality of everyday life as described by Berger and Luckman (1991) in an attempt to address the objective-subjective split that has provoked centuries of philosophical debate and continues its dogged pursuit into the social sciences. It relates to what is reality and how can one know it. Setting aside much of the historical unresolvable theorising within the sociology of knowledge, Peter Berger 1990, P20–24 focus's on the knowledge that constitutes the fabric of meanings without which society would disintegrate[4] and so too would the sanity of individuals caught in a meaningless or anomic world.

Society may have an observable and measurable 'objective facticity', but it is also created and recreated by individuals and communities in ways that reflect their subjective world of perceptions, ideas, and beliefs (p. 30).[5] However, while agreeing on the dialectical relationship between an external, objective reality and the individual's subjective experience of it, not all phenomena are universally and similarly perceived or responded to; the cultures, environments, and genetic material that we inherit and inhabit also have a say in this. Across various chapters, I explore the origins and disputed territory that psychiatry as an institution of state is expected to 'police' madness on behalf of other citizens while simultaneously caring for those deemed to be mad.

Chapters 7 and 8 consider how these different and often conflicting roles threaten to undermine the trustworthiness of mental health services in relation to the best interests of the individual. If power and motivation are significant dimension of trust, these may be diverse and complex among the actors involved hospital admission and treatment decisions, requiring a consideration of whose trust matters most. Psychiatry as a medical science has been under constant criticism, not least within its own discipline, about the nature and causes of mental illness and the consequent purpose and treatment of the profession; caring, curing, or controlling. Various social groups, women, working-class people, and sexual and minority ethnic communities have regularly raised their own concerns about the trustworthiness of psychiatry, particularly regarding the institution's legitimation and practice of prejudice. People with lived experience, more generally, have questioned the legitimacy of diagnostic labels and treatments that sometimes do more harm than good. The detention of people designated as mentally ill in itself is often considered by patients as a major violation of trust involved. However, it is usually forgotten, that involuntary detention is a complex action in difficult circumstances, often comprising multiple events and transactions undertaken by various actors. Psychiatry, as represented by mental health professionals, assumes the symbolic responsibility and the blame for events that have their origins elsewhere.

Chapter 9 provides an exploration of stigma – how boundaries are erected between people and groups through variation in the interpretation of reality, what constitutes sanity, and who gets to decide where the boundaries lie. Whatever the origins of the phrase 'Whom the gods would destroy, they first make mad', the mechanism between loss of reason and madness is usually situated in other losses – the exclusion from normal social routines and connections, the loss of reputation and trustworthiness. Mental illness (or madness as it sometimes still known) in its various forms has probably always existed. Narratives in literature and the cinema are busy with people deemed irrational, regarded by fellow citizens as eccentric, or exhibiting beliefs and behaviours that didn't quite fit in with the expectations of the community. In most narratives, the lives of the 'mad' are depicted as difficult, they don't end well. In some instances, those considered as different are offered a special place in the community, as highly spiritual, possessing insights and visions not available to others; in others, such people were rejected by the community, deemed too unpredictable to have a productive role to have value. Put another way, the mad were considered disruptive, upset the social order, they embodied and created conflict. The potential for dissonance created by such individuals was either accommodation or exclusion, providing deviance within an alternative significance within the community or simply removal through one means or another. These basic social responses remain today in most societies, often in tandem.

In various sections of the book, I have described challenges and failures of trust at various levels of social organisation and which are collectively and personally damaging. How to tackle the twin matters of social conflict and social trust are outside the scope of this book and my own intellectual capacity. The last chapter offers some thoughts on trust repairing and building in mental health services. Psychiatry and mental health services remain in some disarray, partly due to the institutionalised stigma that leaves service provision disastrously underfunded and leaving nugatory space for understanding the origins of patients' suffering and what might help them.

Notes

1   It is important to note a variation in approval levels for different branches of government. Thus, the postal service and the centre for disease control are more trusted, perhaps unsurprisingly, than police and tax services.

2 However, while the word is ubiquitous in everyday communication, the concept is only superficially discussed in everyday life. Many of us will think of it as a feeling, a 'gut instinct', a reaction to someone's past difficult or unpredictable behaviour or their perceived low morality. Because trust assumes a taken for granted existence it seldom provokes much personal interrogation.

3 George Simnel has been credited by Barbara Misztal (2013) and others (Möllering, 2001) as the source of much of our understanding of trust, providing others with the basis for a theoretical framework for personal and generalised trust.

4 In doing so, they acknowledge the influence of George Herbert Mead and later work within American symbolic interactionism. Like Bourdieu's 'structuring structures' of the habitus, Berger and Luckman affirm the dualism in social reality which allows for a dialectical relationship between objectivity and subjectivity.

5 However, while much of the objective facticity of the external world has a commonly apprehended reality, war, or poverty, for example, the reasons for this or that phenomenon are often a battlefield of disputed beliefs and theories. We can acknowledge the ubiquitous use of internet technology in working life but while some might see it as a form of oppressive corporate control, others might it as an efficient form of communication – the challenge of ideology, described by Berger and Luckman.

References

Bateman, A., Brown, D., & Pedder, J. (2000). *Introduction to psychotherapy: An outline of psychodynamic principles and practice*. Routledge.

Beckett, S. (2006). *Waiting for Godot*. Faber & Faber.

Berger, P. L. (1990). *The Sacred Canopy: Elements of a sociological theory of religion*. Random House, pp. 20–24.

Berger, P., & Luckman, T. (1991). *The social construction of reality: A treatise in the sociology of knowledge*. Penguin.

Bourdieu, P. (1977). *Outline of a theory of practice*. Cambridge University Press.

Bowlby, J. (1988). *A secure base*. Routledge.

Camus, A. (2005). *The myth of Sisyphus*. Penguin.

Curran, E., Rosato, M., Ferry, F., & Leavey, G. (2020). Prevalence and factors associated with anxiety and depression in older adults: Gender differences in psychosocial indicators. *Journal of Affective Disorders*, *267*, 114–122. https://doi.org/10.1016/j.jad.2020.02.018

Giddens, A. (1991). *Modernity and self-identity: self and society in the late modern age*. Polity Press.

Littlewood, R., & Lipsedge, M. (1989). *Aliens and alienists* (2nd ed.). Unwin Hyman.

Lyotard, J.-F. (1994). *The postmodern condition*. Manchester.

Misztal, B. (2013). *Trust in modern societies: The search for the bases of social order*. John Wiley & Sons.

Möllering, G. (2001). The nature of trust: From Georg Simmel to a theory of expectation, interpretation and suspension. *Sociology*, *35*, 403–420.

Pilgrim, D., Tomasini, F., & Yassilev, I. (2011). *Examining trust in health care: A multidisciplinary perspective*. Palgrave Macmillan.

Reemtsma, J. P. (2012). *Trust and violence: An essay on a modern relationship*. Princeton University Press.

Swidler, A. (1986). Culture in action: Symbols and strategies. *American Sociological Review*, *51*(2), 273–286. https://doi.org/10.2307/2095521

Taylor, C. (2021). The politics of recognition. In *Campus wars* (pp. 249–263). Routledge.

Vigo, D., Thornicroft, G., & Atun, R. (2016). Estimating the true global burden of mental illness. *Lancet Psychiatry*, *3*(2), 171–178. https://doi.org/10.1016/s2215-0366(15)00505-2

Chapter 2

Social Dimensions of Trust

The literature on trust has been focussed mostly on the mechanisms of integration – how to minimise friction and conflict within society and between citizens and institutions. For economists, understanding the dynamics and determinants of trust is regarded as crucial to the efficient planning and running of organisations. For government, trust is central to policy to minimise conflict between communities or between citizens and government for notions concerned with the 'national good'. Most prominent among sociologists with a renewed interest in trust, Anthony Giddens (1991) explored its significance in relation to risk within the contexts of modernity and the emergence of complex, abstract systems, taking into account that modern societies are subject to rapid, often unanticipated change. Given the rapidly changing global economic landscape, and high levels of international instability, the need to understand trust, if anything, has become more relevant. It is reasonable to suggest that the concept of trust was never a dominating topic in the social sciences let alone the sociology of health. George Simnel has been credited (Misztal, 2013; Möllering, 2001) as the source of much of our understanding of trust, providing others with the basis for a theoretical framework for the conceptualisation of personal and generalised trust. Misztal (2013, pp. 2–3) noted a recent shift in the disciplinary exploration of trust from relatively narrow disputes about institutional confidence in states and markets no longer regarded as merely a 'regulatory mechanism but rather as a public good' with much wider contributions to our understanding of trust in social policy, community relations, conflict, and health.

Of interest to governments and social commentators alike is an age of individualism and the rapid decline of belief systems and institutions what will now help bind people into a community. From whence will integration and cohesion emerge in a pluralist world of atomised self-interest. In this perspective, it is not just civil society that is threatened but the future of community, the totality of connections that constitute mutual (and moral) obligations and responsibilities which trust produces and reproduces. Of additional significant concern is the volume of distrust, hostility, and alienation towards democratic processes, the growth of intolerance, and extremism. These provoke conflicting responses as to what constitutes progress, national and personal identity, individual freedoms, and collective responsibility. Enlightenment hopes of human progress and peace through rational,

DOI: 10.4324/9781003326687-2

scientific knowledge seem rather optimistic, to say the least. Savage, intensely violent conflict across most continents shows few signs of subsiding, coupled with the increasingly destructive impacts produced by climate change, bringing new levels of anxiety to our populations.

However, community cohesion and trust are also dynamic, influenced by events at the national and local levels.[1] Thus, while there are similar challenges to social cohesion across Western nations and regions, there are also major distinctions shaped by historical forces and determinants. These may be ethnic or sectarian divisions that are legacies of colonialism or economic disparities across regions. Whatever their origin, conflict has severe and enduring impacts on community wellbeing and on the mental health of individuals.

In the following sections, I set out some of the definitions, contours, and applications of trust, beginning with social trust. The concept of trust remains ambivalent and ill-defined because of its application in heterogenous, often distinct contexts and disciplines. Thus, while trust between business organisations may share some similar essential or foundational trust characteristics as interpersonal relationships, more emotional dimensions of the latter suggest different trust outcomes and approaches. The citizen's disposition in trusting politicians and the political system is different to that of the citizen as patient towards healthcare and physicians. Moreover, additional complexity arises from the characteristics and dispositions of both the trustee and trustor. Various sociodemographic characteristics (e.g. sex, social class, ethnicity, and age, among others) contain the potential bases for power and vulnerability. There is therefore some need to disentangle the concept of trust and its respective relevance for mental health across interpersonal, general, and organisational domains. Specifically, not only must we consider the making and breaking of trust and its relationship with mental health at the social and personal levels but also the significance of those tasked with resolving and repairing. While the conceptualisation of trust remains problematic and requires considerable unpacking, others have suggested that the idea of trust as an essential and positive force in society is often exaggerated (Cook & Gerbasi, 2012). As discussed in various chapters, the role of trust and its construction within social capital and in healthcare should be treated with some caution.

Overcoming uncertainty

Without general trust, it is argued that much of human life in all its infinite operations would likely grind to halt or, at least, become grindingly difficult, tedious, and impact on health and wellbeing. As Simmel suggests, relationships endure because trust carries more weight than 'rational proof or personal observation'. If it where otherwise, most religions would have never persisted as long as they have or ever have taken root. Reduced social complexity, social cohesion, order, and the ability to govern are all predicated, to some degree, on trust. Without it, life might become uncertain, complicated, and tiresome, to say the least. Without trust, every negotiation with individuals and organisations would be tedious, mired in anxiety, hesitation, and endless verification. The spontaneity of interdependence in every-day would wither substituted with tedious bureaucratic monitoring and endless, costly legal controls.

Trust is a solution, albeit a partial one, to the challenges of uncertainty. If the outcome of a particular action or engagement is predictable, trust does not enter the equation. The increasing unpredictability of modernity and reliance on abstract systems, relative to the simplicity of social relations and expectations that obtained in pre-modern societies, creates a greater role for trust as a mechanism to man-age uncertainty and risk (Luhmann, 1988). Thus, the complexity of modern life demands mechanisms (in Luhmann's terms, generalised media) that facilitate trust and in so doing, reduces complexity or rather, the individual's negotiation of com-plexity by transcending poor knowledge and offering a sense of security instead (Luhmann, 1979). However, trust in the 'system' cannot be assumed as a universal or permanent fixture but is predicated on context and the individual's confidence. As we later discuss on the personal foundations of trust, individuals are more likely to trust from a position of self-confidence – that they are more willing to be vul-nerable in a situation with others if they feel able to manage risk and disappoint-ment. Less emphasis is given in the trust literature to Luhmann's recognition of the importance of mistrust as a mechanism for security (1979, p. 75). Operationalised when appropriate rather than the default response mistrust can be healthy but as we note in later sections, mistrust can tip over into the pathological for society and the individual, and easily weaponised by bad actors.

In this, Barbalet (2009) emphasises not only trust's value and its fragility to deception but also its lack of protection. Trust may open the portal for engage-ment and action but ultimately is no guarantor of a desirable outcome for those who depend on or seek it. Resonant of Weber's description of bureaucratic control, modern organisations strive to establish and maintain regularity in relationships, therefore minimising reliance on trust. Lacking omnipotence, organisations cannot control all the moving parts within their own environments nor influence change in external environments – political, cultural, or economic – although powerful organisations attempt to do so.

Modern organisational systems and processes, whether these are financial or healthcare, are increasingly complex. Where once connection and communication between 'consumers' and 'service providers' were direct and personal, exchange between individuals and organisations is indirect and impersonal, often mediated through non-human processes using artificial intelligence and guided by algo-rithms. While rationality may be simultaneously be an organisational ideal and strategy, and the employees within complex sectors tightly constrained in their actions and relationship, they remain human all the same. Emotions, motivations, and beliefs can always threaten to resist the best efforts of technical and bureau-cratic systems. And, while organisational control systems may appear rigid and of-fer a sense of certainty, leadership, and systems are prone to change. A predictable outcome yesterday is not guaranteed tomorrow. Moreover, trust is not a substitute for control. There is a voluntary surrender of control from those who trust, an acceptance of dependency on the other party, while also acknowledging the potentiality for betrayal, usually entailing the loss of something of value. The importance of the object of value (e.g. health, dignity, money, and love) determines the measure of trust, what is at stake, and the impact of betrayal. The other key defining and intertwined dimension of trust, common to all contexts, is its future orientation and unknowability; into this 'black box' of limited knowledge, to trust is to place a kind of 'blind faith' in the desired outcome.

The connection between choice and trust is problematic and requires more discussion. As other commentators have indicated, trust is irrelevant in the context of coercion. It cannot be argued that an individual's trust is activated towards the achievement of a goal when the action is forced upon them. However, where choices are available between different agencies, and there is a preference for one over the others, the choice may signal trust but can also resemble something closer to a gamble when knowledge is equally unobtainable for all possible choice options. Nevertheless, while a complicating factor, the potential for choice between alternative options, leaves trust intact – we cannot know that we have made the correct decision in the placing of trust until a future desirable outcome has been obtained or thwarted.

A longstanding distinction has been the conceptualisation of human beings as either essentially cooperative or competitive. Famously, Thomas Hobbes (2016) viewed the latter as determining human behaviour and relationships. Trust, commonly associated with wellbeing and security, is more likely to produce efficient cooperation and when weak or absent, daily existence can be experienced as precarious. Often a taken-for-granted condition, trust permits relatively swift exchange of goods and free passage of people. Linked as it is, with vulnerability, distrust, conversely, tends to mire individuals and communities in a demanding process of examination and verification; vulnerability is in an inverse relationship to trust. Trust, therefore, is often characterised as kind of latent glue that binds social members, a central component within the social cohesion and the threat to it, that Putnam (2000) raised in his highly influential book *Bowling Alone*. Due to the interconnectedness and interdependence of close relationships, the risk of betrayal is minimised but remains possible. As in all groups, emergent cultural rules that regulate relationships and activities become reified, assuming 'natural' and enduring properties inherited across generations. As with organisational and bureaucratic processes, culture helps ensure, or at least attempts to bind, community members to levels of conformity which drives much of the predictability in social behaviour. In doing so, culture, custom, and tradition reduce the contingency and precariousness that are prior conditions for the existence of trust, removing rather than resolving the problem to which trust may be a solution (Barbalet, 2009). However, such conceptions of culture suggest it as containing somewhat static and stultifying qualities, whereby beliefs and behaviours are impervious to change and adaptability.

Most communities, even those rigidly religion-based, are susceptible to variation in cultural shifts, charismatic leaders, and schism, commonly a mixture of internal and external influences. Thus, change happens in tight-knit communities but in comparison with more open and permeable secular communities, perhaps more glacially. Thus, the mainstream faiths have continually fragmented over centuries and will continue to do so. While old certainties can dissolve rapidly, trust remains a solution to uncertainty wrought by cultural change. However, in accepting trust's role in maintaining predictability, trust also preserves custom and denies change. Thus, the preservation of trustworthy community membership is embedded in the individual meeting the expectation of others as the failure to do so may provoke a loss of respect and a loss or diminution in the quality or quantity of relationships. Because the loss of bonds can be universally damaging, integrity is maintained with minimal membership attrition. The potential for sanctions provides further assurance of trust and the resistance to default on the expectation.

While social capital within tightly-knit communities may appear to be strong, such communities are preserved through the exclusion of 'outsiders'. The preservation of one's own community is also maintained by the belief, whether tacitly or explicitly propagated, that there is a superiority to protect, an advantage over other communities. The extension of trust to the 'black box' of other communities may represent a dilution of the certainty provided within one's own. The 'narcissism of small difference' in Freud's terms 'a convenient and relatively harmless satisfaction of the inclination to aggression, by means of which cohesion between members of the community is made easier' (1961). Thus, differences between communities may be marginal, often undetectable to other outsiders, but are highly valued by the insiders and which establish a mutual sense of strangeness and antipathy giving rise to various expressions of conflict. In settings where community difference appear to dissolve, violence is often summoned to re-establish differences (Figlio, 2018). Symbolic boundaries are described by Lamont and Molnar as 'conceptual distinctions made by social actors to categorise objects, people, practices, and even time and space'. Such distinctions are settled over time by groups to define reality, providing 'alternative systems and principles of classifications'. Concurrent with defining an alternative understanding of reality, symbolic boundaries provide a commonality of identify and belonging (Lamont & Molnar, 2002). Social boundaries are essential elements of social structures determining resources and social opportunities. Formed after the establishment of symbolic boundaries, social boundaries begin to create recognisable forms of separation and exclusion, membership, relationships, and roles.

Routinisation and predictability

Even in totalitarian societies, human behaviour tends to be guided and shaped by innumerable micro-laws, generalised environmental expectations of how things are, and what will happen given this or that action. The routinisation of life is usually determined within a particular set of cultural norms – polite behaviour in restaurants, orderly queuing at bus stops, or that our neighbours can be expected not to park their car in our driveway or invade our homes. Sometimes these expectations are underwritten by legislation – driving on the wrong side of the road or beating up one's children (or someone else's) tends to be frowned upon in most societies, to varying degrees. International legislation and courts have been established in the hope of maintaining order or punishing transgression. Nevertheless, our implicit faith in that we will experience no harm or suffer a negative consequence in the undertaking of daily activities permits the free continuance of interactions with the environment and relationships. However, we can only discuss this level of trust in generalities; a desired state produced within ideal conditions. People and nations behave badly, traffic lights break down. Other actions that develop and bolster trust between individuals and their environment break down too, or never existed.

Misztal (2013, p. 111) suggests that 'we are trapped into the web of habit, even when we try to develop means of protection against routinised practices or when we try to liberate ourselves from the power of unreflective forces'. Such patterns of reflectiveness on ritualistic behaviours only become apparent in collision with external events such as a trauma, violence, bereavement, or illness which often force a re-examination of past and future life. The routinisation and ritualism of everyday life is a defence against anxiety, not only bolstering ontological security but also facilitates inertia and the stultification of creativity and change. More problematically perhaps, routinisation may also promote behaviours considered dangerous, unethical, or immoral. Thus, routinisation of practice and custom in healthcare can act as a barrier to the introduction of evidence-based practices and the removal of harmful clinical processes. Unreflective routinisation may also provide individuals and groups with moral reassurance in the undertaking of racist or other discriminatory acts, until disrupted and challenged. The formation of ideological 'knowledge' that emerge from routinisation within general social worlds are transmitted to and supported by other spheres, actively or passively. Thus, religio-cultural beliefs regarding human sexuality were for many years readily absorbed into standard psychiatric knowledge and classificatory systems. For some people, the hyper-routinisation of habit may be transformed into behaviours that are considered by others as pathological. Most of us can be located on a spectrum of socially acceptable behaviours of one kind or another. For example, an individual's need for cleanliness and hygiene may stray into a barrier to normal functioning and diagnose as an obsessional compulsive disorder, a fear of being out of control and a maladaptive defence against the anxiety this creates. Most of us tolerate the idiosyncratic behaviour of others until they interfere with the equilibrium of our worlds, then they become a problem; however, such problems may be classified.

Again, we need to distinguish between trust and confidence as concepts – and these might be critical in negotiating trust as a personal quality. I might be confident in a professional's skills and abilities, but I may not trust them to deal with me honestly. Again, I might not trust the person in authority, but it would be of considerable benefit to me if she/he were able to overcome whatever biases they hold and begin to trust me. Here, we acknowledge that trust is bi-directional and dynamic. Not a static trait or attitude of one individual but constructed dialectically, even if in the act of the construction, there is a high degree of inauthenticity. I need your trust in order to fulfil certain needs – it requires me to behave in a certain way, present in ways that are not usual to me but are acceptable to you. In healthcare, as in most other institutions and services, the ability to engage, negotiate, and obtain trust can be crucial to a favourable outcome. An individual's ability to negotiate is developed in early childhood and may be predicated not only on the occurrence of adverse events but also on more subtle cues and resources in the environment.

Various commentators (Granovetter, 1983; Hardin, 2006; Misztal, 2013) have distinguished between categories of 'thin' trust and 'thick' trust, the former a development of modern societies and typically found at the institutional level, usually underpinned by bureaucratic legalism. 'Thick' trust is considered to be that which is found in community and kinship, that is, it thickens over time through increased contact and familiarity. However, friendship networks in modernity are no longer restricted by locale or religious beliefs and organisations; they can be constructed and maintained through diverse institutions and mechanisms of interest and activity. Associations and groups based on aspects of identity that matter to the individual are formed and may flourish over time and space. There is the potential and opportunity too for long-term commitment or ephemeralness. Indeed, various modern organisations have attempted to nurture qualities of 'thick' trust among staff, emphasising virtues of loyalty, teamwork, and commitment, whereby the workplace milieu comes to be 'a second family'.

Several factors or conditions provide the basis for trust. First, within contractual relationships, whether these are community based or commercial, past experience in the form of personal knowledge and familiarity provide the basis of predictability and the level of trust that may be assumed. Second, trust in a weak form may be guaranteed through a third party, an authority such as a government agency who may sanction against breaches of trust. In a developed society with strong legal frameworks, if the goods I buy from the shopkeeper are faulty, regardless of any inconvenience, I may be reimbursed. In a society lacking such legal sanctions, a habitual defaulter may face direct community boycott, unless he/she is in a monopolistic position. In this context, trust is only partially relevant since the actions of the bad agent can be remedied. Nevertheless, the shopper may feel that trust has been betrayed if they have been a regular customer and established a familiarity.

Trust exists and thickens through dialectical mechanisms, feedback loops which expose individuals to other individuals and then deepens through continued contact. The longer the individual's expectations within a relationship are fulfilled, or at least not betrayed, the more likely that trust will be maintained. If the level of interpersonal trust is low, continued contact is unlikely. Trust-building also thrives through reciprocity. At increasing levels of intimacy, individuals may self-disclose evidence of personal vulnerability which may then require an equivalent token of vulnerability. However, contained within any feedback loop, there is always the potential for the disappointment of trust and a deterioration in contact and experience.

Generalised trust

Although much of what is written about trust concerns the functional properties of the concept of generalised trust (Möllering, 2001), there is no consensus on its value. Bizarrely perhaps, given it is the basis of myriad national and international surveys which purport to tap into the wellbeing of our social and democratic institutions by examining our trust relationships with non-specific others in society. Thus, survey respondents are required to state the extent to which they believe that people are trustworthy most of the time. The political scientist, Russell Hardin is scathing about the value of such questions by offering the response that one can only assess the people that one most frequently deals with most of the time, not lots of others whom one wouldn't trust, most of the time, or might simply be 'agnostic' about their trustworthiness (Hardin, 2006, p. 124). Hardin suggests that what is taken as 'generalised trust' is little more than simple optimism about the cooperativeness of one's fellow citizens, to which most of us can attest, most of the time. But it is the lack of specificity of persons and contexts that is crucial to the undermining of the notion of generalised trust. Though many people have placed their trust in people who then fleece them of all their savings, this is a process not an event. As just another confidence 'trick' the perpetrator takes time to build a relationship, identifying the victim's vulnerabilities, which often include loneliness. In the absence of some cognitive impairment or other, people do not hand over large sums of money to strangers. What is taken as generalised trust must then rest on a general disposition towards others. In Hardin's example, a child who has emerged into adulthood from a relatively 'benign environment' in which trustworthiness was the norm is more likely to have 'relatively positive expectations by inductive generalization' (Hardin, 2006, p. 126), a view similar to Luhmann's understanding of the individual's self-confidence in relation to a general disposition to trust.

Hardin's negative assessment of the concept of generalised trust is convincing. If we cannot plausibly offer blanket appraisal of trustworthiness in society, it is more likely that our generalised judgements are based on stereotyping based on characteristics or qualities perceived to be held by this or that group but not others that they may be sufficiently trustworthy in a particular situation or context. A lone female may be reasonably comfortable in sharing a car with a group of other women but maybe more likely to decline the offer from a group of male footballers. In the absence of other useful information, stereotype-based decision-making has a pragmatic logic even though we might argue that it is inherently wrong. Allowing for the fact that stereotypes can be positive as well as negative and how one assesses the direction may depend on your relationship to the group being stereotyped. If a religious community or political party broadcast views that are considered by misogynistic or racist it is reasonable to anticipate a challenging relationship with the membership if you happen to be a woman or a migrant. Generalised distrust in such cases is a rational response in specific contexts.

Problematically, if the notion of generalised trust is of questionable value, then what is it that is being measured within studies hoping to measure it? We may assume that most survey respondents believed the question of the general trustworthiness of people to be sensible. The survey response rates suggest that this is so. In addition to the person's individual disposition to trust or mistrust generated by life experience, the survey data may be telling us something about feelings of ambient connectedness, and/or safety, that people in the broader society are generally well-meaning, not criminally minded. Their response to 'generalised trust' questions may point to general political-philosophical dispositions, a view that humans are either best represented by Hobbes or Rousseau.

Problematically too, interests can be differently defined by parties with similar goals. In many instances, we can never truly know that both parties will have full agreement on the nature of the 'best interests'. Even where a generally amicable or loving relationship exists between two closely related individuals, the actions and desired or expected outcomes by one person may be perceived as bewildering betrayal by the other. My beliefs about my best interests in this immediate situation and time may diverge radically from the beliefs of the other person who sees them best served by another, longer-term, strategy. I may not be able to see the 'bigger picture' envisaged by my loved one, whom I trust usually, but in this matter, feel utterly betrayed. Trust may also rapidly evaporate as events and circumstances change.

Equality, relationships, and power

To the various overarching, national and cultural dimensions of trust may be added inter-communal factors – such as the degree of equality or disparities in a society, the distribution, and access of groups to power and justice. Distilling these dynamics, we start from the rather prosaic acknowledgement that economic and social differences produce consequent inequalities in relation to needs, goods, and interests across different groups which are differentially met through power – the ability of an individual (or group) to influence another in the pursuit of a particular outcome through, sometimes against the wishes or interests of the other. It is in this relationship that trust is most easily recognised. Power has various dimensions or characteristics that relate to trust, negatively or positively. Thus, the concept of trust is irrelevant in a relationship of coercive power is and the action towards a goal provides no alternatives or options. In other expressions of power, it doesn't matter if person B is generally regarded as acting collaboratively with person A; legitimate power presents as a more tacit acceptance of the other person's 'superior' position in an organisational hierarchy and their expectation of being 'in control' of others' behaviours towards organisational goals. In places, this power can extend to the expressed attitudes, dress code, and, increasingly in modern bureaucratic organisations, the prohibition of personal relationships particularly where these, ironically perhaps, include power differentials. As we shall discuss, power, hierarchical position, and autonomy are associated with trust, and health and wellbeing outcomes.

Inequality and trust

In the United Kingdom, the early lockdown policy was manifestly successful – mostly, people stayed at home, social distanced, and wore masks. Moreover, there was an outpouring of social solidarity, particularly directed at frontline workers in health and social care. Despite the hardships and personal privations, there was a consensus in most Western societies that government was acting in the best interests of the nation as a whole – in the words of an oft quoted political slogan, 'we're all in it together!'. Except, of course, that the collective and egalitarian virtues signalled in the message were eventually exposed as false. Some communities were more impacted by COVID 19 than others. Black and minority ethnic communities, older people in care homes, and the financially disadvantaged experienced much higher rates of morbidity and mortality than their counterparts in the general population. While many people lost their jobs and livelihoods, others benefited financially. As the pandemic progressed, media stories emerged how individuals and companies, often connected to government politicians, made inordinate profits selling dubious or useless goods or services. Later still, it was revealed that the government disregarded lockdown rules that they imposed on its citizens, misbehaved in various illegal celebrations, and then lied to parliament and the population. It is not hard to detect the key aspects of trust and its erosion in social and political systems. First, an expectation that another party (government) will have the best interests of all citizens in mind in making and implementing policy. This includes an expectation that the sacrifice is shared and no one person or group will benefit, and this includes those who make the rules. Second, the sense of betrayal of trust is commensurate with the demands and the sacrifices made. An innate belief in equality and a sense of unfairness about inequalities is deeply entwined with trust and mistrust, playing a role, it is argued, in the occurrence and effects of anomie – including poor health, violence and social conflict, and mental illness.

Social capital and trust

The exigencies arising from the COVID pandemic and the public health measures accelerated the dynamics of disembedding – technology now permits the possibility of living in Cambodia while working for a New York company, for example. The massive social rupture created by the pandemic with its rapid abandoning of past shibboleths and practices continues to reveal the fragility of tradition and habit. The implications for the organisation of work, our city centres, and domestic relations may have changed forever. The shift towards secularism in many Western societies, consumerism, and the cultural hypermarket that the internet permits has disembedded these social relations faster and more extensively than most institutions can feel comfortable with. Not simply religious organisations and governments, of course, many groups and communities feel unable to cope with the speed and direction of change in modern societies.

The nature of modern institutions and our relationship with them has become increasingly tenuous and problematic, producing both ontological and social concerns among citizens about the location and direction of power and authority, agency and control, human value, and truth. Giddens is clear that modern institutions are a radical departure from previous forms of social order in the way that they 'undercut traditional habits and customs'. We can go further and argue that while modern institutions challenge and disrupt traditions, the reverse can also be true. However, writing at the infancy of the internet and long before the ubiquity of the algorithm and the anxiety created by artificial intelligence, Giddens (1991) could not have predicted the social dominance and the unrestrained wealth of tech companies, the speed of globalisation, the diffusion of information dislocated from fact, and the impotence of sovereign governments to regulate the spread of disinformation and divisiveness. In the flow of dynamic change, these dimensions of modernity continue to have profound implications for the individual and society arising from uncertainties of self-identity and belonging, and where truth and trust may be ascertained. In a pre-modern existence, unless conscripted into an army, most people lived and died in the same town or village, accepted the existence of one true faith, viscerally understood clearly where power came from, and possessed a clear understanding of right and wrong, regardless of their adherence to such. For Giddens, modern social life is distinguished from previous eras by a reorganisation of time and space and the presence of 'disembedding mechanisms' that alter social relations that were once tethered to specific locales. Individuals are no longer confined by local needs and traditions but have the freedom (or arguably compelled) to flexibly relocate. Certainly, the relocation of the individual from one distinct cultural locale to another culturally different milieu has implications for the belief systems of the migrant and the host – at the very least there is the potential for multiculturalism to undermine certainties of values and behaviours.

Culture and structure

Bourdieu's theory on cultural and social capital may help us consider some of the mechanisms that determine differences between working, and middle-class individuals in decision-making and health behaviour (cultural capital), and their skills at trust-management in their relationships with professionals (social capital). Cultural capital has been defined as a set of social norms, values, tastes, relational behaviours, aesthetic preferences (e.g. in clothing, food, and art), and so on, which are provided or absorbed through social networks and connections and familial social and institutional contexts within which individuals are embedded (Bourdieu, 1977). Cultural and/or educational capital is manifested in the knowledge, skills, behaviours, and assets of people and regarded as possessing cultural significance by dominant group members. Embodied cultural capital as a form of power and advantage has been linked positively to improved health outcomes and these are intergenerational. Thus, people from disadvantaged backgrounds are likely to have relatively fewer health educational resources than those from middle-class milieu. Likewise, poor health behaviours are more prevalent and less disapproved.

The overlap between cultural and social capital overlap explains the development of trust and quality of relationships with professionals. Social capital, provides a level of compound benefit generated through 'contacts and group memberships which, through the accumulation of exchanges, obligations and shared identities, provide actual or potential support and access to valued resources' (Bourdieu, 1993, p. 143) are also relevant. These resources provide an array of benefits to people from professional and middle-class backgrounds in that they provide access to network contacts among similar others from professional fields. These networks of trustworthy others bring knowledge, expertise, and signposting which facilitate the navigation of usually closed institutions. Building familiarity, and the competencies of negotiation, with professionals and agencies at an early age allows for the generation of trust with these groups and the willingness to seek support from similar professionals in other situations and circumstances. Importantly, the individual reinforces a strong 'locus of control' or agency, again with positive impacts on health outcomes. These advantages intersect with other non-health choices and can often be linked to the habitus or the embodied practices and grammar of everyday life which individuals inherit and develop through their social connections and environments.

Bourdieu's *habitus* (1985) is a helpful conceptual lens for the understanding of class-related health behaviour and help-seeking. Thus, there is, potentially, a myriad of culturally informed beliefs about and responses to the symptoms of this or that mental illness. Different social groups approach the world with considerable interpretative variation and dispositions towards health and other phenomena. An individual can reasonably predict the response of his or her family and community to the expression of an illness, for example, with fear, blame, and intolerance, or compassion and care. That is not to suggest that culture is of itself a determining factor. While social networks are networks of meaning, they are not formed independent of objective social structures, but rather they are informed and shaped by material interests (Rubenstein, 2001). While the cultural beliefs attached to mental healthcare in some communities arise simply from considerations of availability and cost, coping responses to adversity and different levels of emotional literacy or knowledge about psychological treatment are also important. Cultural norms and beliefs may influence behaviours about gender and identity, shame, autonomy, stoicism, and endurance. Thus, even within the micro-culture of a family one quickly learns what behaviour is acceptable or not, how distress is responded to by adults – ignored or treated compassionately.

Class and trust

Crucially, cultural practices are malleable, open to opportunistic interpretation 'formulated and reformulated by actors engaged in practical situations that consist, importantly, in the structure of opportunity' (Rubenstein, 2001, p. 12). An individual's economic position constrains what kind of healthcare is available, as well as its quantity and quality, but can also shape his or her beliefs about such options, the usefulness of a particular modality or the characteristics, motivations, and trustworthiness of its practitioners. For example, private psychotherapy, commonly expensive and therefore in the general preserve of more affluent middle classes, is unlikely to be found in poor neighbourhoods but also more likely to be dismissed by the working class as ineffective and its practitioners disparaged as 'out of touch', among other things. But, if many families from poor neighbourhoods cannot afford treatment (Snowden & Thomas, 2000), then psychotherapy or other talking therapies will have no value in that neighbourhood and will not be discussed as an appropriate source of help – without finance and without discussion, *de facto* psychotherapy does not exist.

However, even when working-class people seek psychotherapy, it may not be a level playing field due to a classist bias by therapists. A substantial body of evidence has accumulated on the prejudicial attitudes and behaviours of middle-class professionals towards poor and working-class people. It has been noted that while people who are defined as middle class or affluent experience any number of 'isms' – racism, sexism, ageism, and heterosexism or have been discriminated against because of a disability – they are unlikely to ever personally experience the stigma and exclusion associated with poverty. Lott (2002), a psychologist, concludes that even though some within the 'discipline of psychology may come from a low-income or working-class background, but it is clearly not a salient feature of their current lives'.

Much of the class-based discriminatory activity is based on conscious or unconscious prejudices but, similar to other discrimination, nurtured by recognisable stereotypes of stupidity, brutishness, laziness, violent, chaotic, and that poverty is a self-inflicted state. Such class-based stereotypes are casually embedded in public discourse and given credence by politicians in ways that would be considered unacceptable if applied to other communities. Lott (2001) and colleagues in the United States argue that predominant among these stereotypes of low-income parents held by educators are beliefs about the parent's lack of concern about their children's schooling, incompetence in helping with homework, and their lack of encouragement for academic success. There is a highly damaging sequalae to teacher judgements on the capacity and character of low-income parents that may determine that their children are predestined to failure and therefore any additional teaching is wasted effort. At what point does an individual's mistrust become a symptom of, or a risk factor for, a mental health problem, or conversely. Certainly, low trust, loneliness, and depressed mood are all interconnected, and for some people, these appear to be present across the lifespan, not just situational conditions. If an individual's disposition towards trust were amenable to a therapeutic intervention, would their mental health improve?

Social inequalities, trust, and health

Historically, in many Western societies, mental illnesses were considered as inherited or as both a consequence and a cause of a person's immoral temperament and behaviour; in many instances, the immorality was considered genetic too. Poverty and ill-health were assumed to have the same origins (MacKenzie, 1976). While, early social reformers and epidemiologists, working separately in the 19th century recognised the connections between environmental squalor, poverty, and poor health, suggesting that moral turpitude and madness is more likely to flourish amid absolute poverty, cultural explanations for health disparities prevailed. It is only much later in the 20th century that epidemiologists began to consider the social determinants of health more fully and the possibility that economic disparities (relative, rather than absolute poverty) might be the source of many social ills including criminal behaviour, violence, stress, mental illness, and mortality.

Structural theories of health inequalities argue that alternative explanations are lacking. Thus, culture and life-style behaviours or intelligence may be theorised as mechanisms that connect structural determinants and health outcomes but fail to ascertain the underlying origins of disparities (McCartney et al., 2013). Influenced by Durkheim, social epidemiologists, such as Lisa Berkman et al. (2014), argue that searching for risk factors at the individual level means that potential interventions are restricted inevitably to individual behaviours. With the originating causal factors intact, future cohorts of people inherit the same set of health problems. While poverty is observably a major risk factor for poor health, associated with deficiencies in bad housing, poor diet, and various other adversities, the importance of relative poverty is increasingly acknowledged. Thus, differences found in mortality rates between developed countries may have less to do with socio-economic differences between them, but rather income differentials *within* them. However, while relative economic differences between individuals matter, there is evidence that power and autonomy can also determine health outcomes.

The Whitehall studies by Marmot and colleagues (Marmot et al., 1978; Smith et al., 1990) which examined the health outcomes of civil servants in the United Kingdom provided evidence of a three-fold difference in mortality between employees at different ends of the hierarchy, even after controlling for the usual risk factors of age, smoking, healthcare access, housing, and lifestyle. Into the relative income and social status, of social position, Wilkinson and others argue that issues of relative power and social status, dominance, and subordination rather than material living standards are key determinants of health. While this is an interesting theory, it leaves considerable gaps in the causal chain in that the micro determinants between power relationships and poor health are unidentified. Is the excess morbidity and mortality among subordinate civil servants observed in these studies due to the stress of objectively measurable harder work or the psychological difficulties generated by being under someone else's control, regardless of whether the boss is kind or horrible? Wilkinson supports his psychosocial theory of health inequalities with studies among primates that reveal similar patterns of wellbeing differentiated by position in the hierarchy (Wilkinson, 1996).

Epidemiologists such as Neal Pearce and George Davey Smith (2003) argue that while there is consensus that income inequality is a major contributor to poor health, evidence for its direct influence is flawed. Other evidence suggests that when factors such as unemployment, low rates of health insurance, per capita medical spending, low educational attainment, and ethnicity are taken into account, income inequality as an explanation disappears (Kaplan et al., 1996). Structuralists maintain that the kind of 'social capital' psychosocial explanations offered by Wilkinson (1996) and others misidentify the true source of poor health by suggesting that socio-economic differences affect health through the individual's self-perception of social ranking whereby a

> perceived low position in the social hierarchy produces negative emotions such as shame and distrust, which are then translated into poor health through psycho-neuro-endocrine mechanisms as well as through stress-induced behaviours such as smoking. At the same time, these negative emotions are translated into antisocial behaviour and reduced participation in community organizations.
>
> (quoted from Pearce & Smith, 2003)

Although the Whitehall studies (Marmot et al., 1991) used a longitudinal design, they were not based on life-course data and therefore, unable to identify more important structural factors that exist before birth and continue to gather importance for health afterwards. Thus, various health problems, including stress, attributed to relatively low hierarchical position may have their origins in childhood disadvantage, problems that are unaltered by social mobility. However, although structural theories appear somewhat more convincing than purely psychosocial explanations, it may be unwise to dismiss the explanatory value of the latter completely. Concealed within income differentials, there are likely to be harsher material and environmental factors that are plausibly more stressful for people in lower social echelons and that these have an additive and accumulatively negative impact on pre-existing risk factors.

Trust and cultural and social capital

Pierre Bourdieu applied the concept of 'capital' beyond its usual financial context and monetary value, permitting a wider consideration of the collective range of symbolic and other resources at the disposal of a community. Thus, cultural capital refers to habits and dispositions, tastes, styles, and dress codes that individuals use, consciously or unconsciously, to signify their symbolic status in society, e.g. activities considered highbrow such as opera and ballet attendance. Social capital is the bank of resources produced by, and contained within, a network of social relationships that members of that group or community can draw upon. These resources may be social and psychological supports that people can access at times of need or crisis, or knowledgeable agents who can assist when building careers or gaining contracts; the latter may be termed as 'affinity networks', that is a network of people bound together by similar backgrounds that generally propel them towards normative and shared interests such as moral or political viewpoints. Thus, such relationships are portable, extending beyond the immediate, local, and the personal. For example, ideology-based groups which use internet platforms to develop networks in the pursuance of political aims, non-violent, or otherwise. Putnam, building on Durkheim's insights on social integration, considered the binding and salutogenic effects of social capital within societies and communities – the level and strength of networks, norms, and social trust that produce mutually beneficial connections, cooperation and exchange (Putnam, 1992). The relative presence of social capital have been examined in a wide range of national and neighbourhood level studies, along with their association with various outcomes such as academic achievement, health and wellbeing (Engström et al., 2008; Kawachi et al., 1999), suicide (Recker & Moore, 2016), violence and crime (Sampson et al., 1997), and volunteering (Cheng et al., 2022). The social connections between individuals and groups are visible through active membership within formally constituted, purposefully directed organisations such as trade unions, professional bodies, political parties, or religious groups. Informal connections are those relationships and activities within families, friendships and neighbourhoods, or local communities, to which may be added the ever-burgeoning communities that emerge through internet platforms and which tend to be superficial and low trust.

Alienation

Durkheim's seminal study of suicide (Durkheim, 1897) in which he considered this most individualistic of actions to be due to *anomie*, a normlessness, generated most acutely by the division of labour and rapid social change, both arising from industrialisation. Although Durkheim's conceptualisation of anomie has been disputed, we can allow that it refers to processes of social fragmentation when traditional sources of authority diminish, leaving dysregulated individuals with little or no shared vision or direction.[2] Much of the literature on trust has been focussed on the mechanisms of integration – how to minimise friction and conflict within society and between citizens and institutions. For economists, understanding the dynamics and determinants of trust is regarded as crucial to the efficient planning and running of organisations. For government, questions of trust are central to minimise conflict between communities or between citizens and government for the 'national good'. Given the rapidly changing global economic landscape, and high levels of international instability, the need to understand trust, if anything, has become more relevant. However, it is reasonable to suggest that the concept of trust was never a dominating topic in the social sciences, let alone the sociology of health. George Simnel has been credited by Barbara Misztal (2013) and others (Möllering, 2001) as the source of much of our understanding of trust, providing others with the basis for a theoretical framework for personal and generalised trust. Misztal (2013, pp. 2–3) suggests that in recent years, there has been a shift away from relatively narrow disputes about institutional confidence in states and markets, no longer regarded as merely a 'regulatory mechanism but rather as a public good'. Most prominent among sociologists with a renewed interest in trust, Anthony Giddens explores its significance in relation to risk within the contexts of modernity and the emergence of complex, abstract systems, taking into account that modern societies are subject to rapid, often unanticipated change (1991).

Of interest to governments and social commentators alike is what will substitute for the erosion of pre-modern belief systems and institutions, the fabric that once bound people into a community. From whence will integration and cohesion emerge in a pluralist world of atomised self-interest. In this perspective, it is not just civil society that is threatened but the future of community, the totality of connections that constitute mutual (and moral) obligations and responsibilities which trust produces and reproduces. Of significant concern is the volume of distrust, hostility, and alienation towards democratic processes, the growth of intolerance, and extremism. These provoke conflicting responses as to what constitutes progress, national and personal identity, individual freedoms, and collective responsibility. Enlightenment hopes of human progress and peace through rational, scientific knowledge seem rather optimistic, to say the least. Savage, intensely violent conflict across most continents shows few signs of subsiding, coupled with the increasingly socially and environmentally destructive impacts produced by climate change; they bring new levels of anxiety to our populations.

However, community cohesion and trust are also dynamic, influenced by events at the national and local levels, amply demonstrated by Brexit and the public health response to COVID, for example. Thus, while there are similar challenges to social cohesion across Western nations and regions, there are also major distinctions shaped by historical forces and determinants. These may be ethnic or sectarian divisions that are legacies of colonialism or economic disparities across regions. Whatever their origin, conflict has severe and enduring impacts on community wellbeing and on the mental health of individuals.

Despite a plethora of policy responses, commonly focussed on migration and ethnic diversity, there is no overarching, sustained approach to understanding the processes related to the erosion and repairing of community connectedness and cohesion. While various governmental branches invest in community cohesion, impact measurement is rarely known. Academic interest and capacity building in community cohesion has been hampered by low interdisciplinarity, a highly localised focus, and generally lacking in the longer-term observation of macro and micro determinants of trust and cohesion. Moreover, there is a need to obtain a better understanding of social cohesion as differently experienced and acknowledged by diverse stakeholders. This is crucial to identifying better indicators of cohesion and developing more accurate measures (Fonseca et al., 2019). Often lacking too, is the relative inclusion of marginalised populations and young people in policy discourses, and how digital technology may be harnessed to promote trust and greater community participation.

There are several competing, often overlapping definitions of community cohesion (Fonseca et al., 2019; Maxwell, 1996). Social capital is possibly the most widely used and policy-friendly conceptualisations on cohesion considers the connections among individuals, their social networks, civic participation, and the norms of reciprocity and trustworthiness. Most, social capital definitions however, emphasise relationships between individuals, communities, and the wider society. They also state the importance of contribution within community life to support a sense of belonging. Other key dimensions include a shared vision underpinned by values of equality, tolerance, fairness, and justice.

Some of the factors associated with strong social cohesion include active citizenship whereby individuals seek to participate in civil society, public institutions, the workplace, and political life. Cohesion also requires a secure citizenship which upholds respect for the rule of law while accompanied by equalities in civil, political, social rights, and responsibilities. Trust is an essential and cross-cutting characteristic of social cohesion. When trust is absent or weak, considerable political, economic, and social costs follow. While open and equitable communication between societal actors creates opportunities for trust-building, the mechanisms for doing so are poorly understood.

Too often, debates concerning society and trust are framed as binary positions, individual needs versus social solidarity. However, individual needs and pursuits are not incompatible with community cohesion and interests. Even in collectivist societies, disruptive individuals pursuing a divergent path were capable of bringing beneficial innovation to the community. As social beings, the individual thrives with the support of the community, even in societies that propagate notions of the self-made person. Again, the focus on competition and conflict may be overstated in academic and policy spheres, overshadowing the more positive dynamics that underpin interdependent and mutually beneficial collaborative pathways that people choose to adopt. Thus, in the latter half of the 20th century and beyond, there is a marked endeavour within the social sciences to envisage and thus build a new path towards social cohesion that permits an accommodation between rational calculative perspectives and the value of civil society. The benefits of well-functioning and integrated communities can be found in the prevention of illness and the protection and care of those who become ill. Thus, the psychiatrist Norman Sartorius (2003) makes the point that well-integrated communities and strong social relationships produce less illness and better prognosis for those who experience illness of any kind and at any age. However, he also makes the point that for social capital to work well, it must be based on an equitable flow of transactions between groups in the production of bonding capital (within communities) and bridging capital (between communities). As explored further in later sections, the concept of social capital may have restricted and uneven relevance to different sections of society. In poorer communities, whatever social capital exists is often exhausted in achieving political visibility and survival; social capital in affluent communities produces more influence and comfort. Again, while social capital might assist in raising social justice and improving the quality of life for the 'general population' in communities, other groups such as those living with severe mental illness remain invisible and disconnected from improvements in community assets.

Notes

1 In the United Kingdom, amply demonstrated by Brexit, and worldwide by terrorism or the COVID pandemic, for example.
2 Later theorists of the 20th century such as Bourdieu explored the concept of social capital, non-monetary resources such as networks that assist individual goals.

References

Barbalet, J. (2009). A characterization of trust, and its consequences. *Theory and Society*, *38*(4), 367–382. http://www.jstor.org/stable/40345659

Berkman, L. F., Kawachi, I., & Glymour, M. M. (eds.) (2014). *Social epidemiology*, 2nd ed. Oxford University Press. https://doi.org/10.1093/med/9780195377903.001.0001

Bourdieu, P. (1977). *Outline of a theory of practice*. Cambridge University Press.

Bourdieu, P. (1985). The forms of social capital. In J. G. Richardson (Ed.), *The handbook of theory and research for the sociology of education* (pp. 241–258). Greenwood.

Bourdieu, P. (1993). *The field of cultural production*. Cambridge University Press.

Cheng, G. H., Chan, A., Østbye, T., & Malhotra, R. (2022). The association of human, social, and cultural capital with prevalent volunteering profiles in late midlife. *European Journal of Ageing*, *19*(1), 95–105. https://doi.org/10.1007/s10433-021-00605-x

Cook, K., & Gerbasi, G. (2012). Trust. In P. Hedström & P. Bearman (Eds.), *The Oxford handbook of analytical sociology* (pp. 218–268). Oxford University Press.

Durkheim, E. (1897). *Suicide*. The Free Press reprint 1997.

Engström, K., Mattsson, F., Järleborg, A., & Hallqvist, J. (2008). Contextual social capital as a risk factor for poor self-rated health: A multilevel analysis. *Social Science & Medicine*, *66*(11), 2268–2280. https://doi.org/10.1016/j.socscimed.2008.01.019

Figlio, K. (2018). The dread of sameness: Social hatred and Freud's "narcissism of minor differences". In *Psychoanalysis and politics* (pp. 29–46). Routledge.

Fonseca, X., Lukosch, S., & Brazier, F. (2019). Social cohesion revisited: A new definition and how to characterize it. *Innovation: The European Journal of Social Science Research*, *32*(2), 231–253. https://doi.org/10.1080/13511610.2018.1497480

Freud, S. (1961). *Civilisation and its discontents*. W. W. Norton.

Giddens, A. (1991). *Modernity and self-identity: Self and society in the late modern age*. Polity Press.

Granovetter, M. (1983). The strength of weak ties: A network theory revisited. *Sociological Theory*, *1*, 201–233. https://doi.org/10.2307/202051

Hardin, R. (2006). *Trust*. Polity.

Hobbes, T. (2016). Leviathan. In *Democracy: A reader* (pp. 37–42). Columbia University Press.

Kaplan, G. A., Pamuk, E. R., Lynch, J. W., Cohen, R. D., & Balfour, J. L. (1996). Inequality in income and mortality in the United States: Analysis of mortality and potential pathways. *BMJ*, *312*(7037), 999–1003. https://doi.org/10.1136/bmj.312.7037.999

Kawachi, I., Kennedy, B. P., & Glass, R. (1999). Social capital and self-rated health: A contextual analysis. *American Journal of Public Health*, *89*(8), 1187–1193. https://doi.org/10.2105/ajph.89.8.1187

Lamont, M., & Molnar, V. (2002). The study of boundaries in the social sciences. *Annual Review of Sociology*, *28*, 167–195. https://doi.org/10.1146/annurev.soc.28.110601.141107

Lott, B. (2001). Low-income parents and the public schools. *Journal of Social Issues, 57*(2), 247–259. https://doi.org/10.1111/0022-4537.00211

Lott, B. (2002). Cognitive and behavioral distancing from the poor. *American Psychologist, 57*, 100–110.

Luhmann, N. (1979). *Trust and power*. Wiley.

Luhmann, N. (1988). Familiarity, confidence, trust: Problems and alternatives. In D. Gambetta (Ed.), *Trust: Making and breaking cooperative relations* (pp. 94–107). University of Oxford.

MacKenzie, D. (1976). Eugenics in Britain. *Social Studies of Science, 6*(3/4), 499–532. http://www.jstor.org/stable/284693

Marmot, M. G., Davey-Smith, G., Stansfeld, S., Patel, C., North, F., Head, J., White, I., Brunner, E., & Feeney, A. (1991). Health inequalities among British civil servants: The Whitehall II study. *Lancet, 337*, 1387–1393.

Marmot, M. G., Rose, G., Shipley, M., & Hamilton, P. J. (1978). Employment grade and coronary heart disease in British civil servants. *Journal of Epidemiology & Community Health, 32*(4), 244–249.

Maxwell, J. (1996). *Social dimensions of economic growth*. Department of Economics, University of Alberta.

McCartney, G., Collins, C., & Mackenzie, M. (2013). What (or who) causes health inequalities: Theories, evidence and implications? *Health Policy, 113*(3), 221–227. https://doi.org/10.1016/j.healthpol.2013.05.021

Misztal, B. (2013). *Trust in modern societies: The search for the bases of social order*. John Wiley & Sons.

Möllering, G. (2001). The nature of trust: From Georg Simmel to a theory of expectation, interpretation and suspension. *Sociology, 35*, 403–420.

Pearce, N., & Smith, G. D. (2003). Is social capital the key to inequalities in health? *American Journal of Public Health, 93*(1), 122–129. https://doi.org/10.2105/ajph.93.1.122

Putnam, R. D. (1992). *Making democracy work: Civic traditions in modern Italy*. Princeton University Press.

Putnam, R. D. (2000). *Bowling alone: The collapse and revival of American community*. Simon and Shuster.

Recker, N. L., & Moore, M. D. (2016). Durkheim, social capital, and suicide rates across US counties. *Health Sociology Review, 25*(1), 78–91. https://doi.org/10.1080/14461242.2015.1101703

Rubenstein, D. (2001). *Culture, structure and agency: Toward a truly multidimensional sociology*. Sage.

Sampson, R. J., Raudenbush, S. W., & Earls, F. (1997). Neighborhoods and violent crime: A multilevel study of collective efficacy. *Science, 277*(5328), 918–924. https://doi.org/10.1126/science.277.5328.918

Sartorius, N. (2003). Social capital and mental health. *Current Opinion in Psychiatry, 16*, S101–S105. https://journals.lww.com/co-psychiatry/fulltext/2003/04002/social_capital_and_mental_health.15.aspx

Smith, G. D., Shipley, M. J., & Rose, G. (1990). Magnitude and causes of socioeconomic differentials in mortality: Further evidence from the Whitehall study. *Journal of Epidemiology & Community Health, 44*(4), 265–270.

Snowden, L. R., & Thomas, K. (2000). Medicaid and African American outpatient mental health treatment. *Mental Health Services Research, 2*(2), 115–120. https://doi.org/10.1023/a:1010161222515

Wilkinson, R. (1996). *Unhealthy societies: The afflictions of inequality*. Routledge.

Chapter 3

Conflict and Trust

Social cohesion, order, and co-operation are predicated on trust, without which the activities of life become uncertain, complicated, tiresome, and potentially injurious; every negotiation with individuals and organisations tediously mired in anxiety, hesitation, and endless verification. Spontaneity would wither, replaced by bureaucratic monitoring, and endless legal and costly controls. It is in this space that we touch upon arguably the most central of all sociological preoccupations – the maintenance of order and the consequences of its failure and then dissolution into conflict. The threat to identity and sense of reality through 'nomic disruption' described by Berger and Luckman (1966) can be applied equally to individual and collective anomic states. Through conflict and violence, the everyday is thrown into a terrorising chaos and potentially, the emptying out of an assumed trust in and between communities. The closer to the universality of violence in any given society, the closer to the destruction of an assumed social reality for all citizens. The kind of collective madness witnessed in total wars.

The World Health Organisation declares that violence is a public health problem (Krug et al., 2002) not only inflicting a heavy toll on the physical and mental health of populations but on the interpersonal relationships that sustain health and healthcare infrastructures. Simmel (1955, p. 13) poses a somewhat paradoxical question when suggesting that conflict 'irrespective of any phenomena that result from conflict or that accompany it, itself is a form of sociation', an engagement with others. It also appears to strengthen community bonding through social solidarity (Durkheim, 1897) by redirecting attention to external threats and in so doing, overshadowing, or at least bracketing internal schisms and factional disputes. Violence as an instrument of conflict, according to Hannah Arendt, is 'rational to the extent that it is effective in reaching the end that must justify it. And since we can never know with any certainty the eventual consequences of what we are doing violence can remain rational only if it pursues short-time goals' (1970, p. 79). Thus, violence and interpersonal conflict, like poor health, are not evenly distributed in society. Nor is trust. If material success is a commonly valued social goal but legitimate opportunities for its attainment are limited, 'deviant' methods offer an alternative route (Merton, 1968). Access denied to scarce and desirable resources or claims may lead to frustration and violence. As noted previously, relatively low

DOI: 10.4324/9781003326687-3

hierarchical power and locus of control means that the destruction may be internally, as well as externally directed.

It is beyond the scope of this (or perhaps any) book to explore the origins and trajectories of conflict, they are all miserable but miserable in their own way, to paraphrase Tolstoy. However, in this chapter, I explore conflict and its relationships with trust as variegated and existing along a continuum. At the milder end, the term can suggest a difference of opinion or belief between individuals or groups. Depending on the closeness of the actors and what is at stake, such conflicts are typically contained and managed by social rules and norms, and easily resolved. Further along the continuum, conflict is expressed as a wide range of challenging behaviours with more problematic consequences, such as domestic violence and family breakup. At the other end, differences between communities or states may escalate to sporadic violence or outright war. I argue that while conflict has the potential to damage and dysregulate body and mind, violence is often an expression of anxiety and mistrust whatever the object of these emotions might be, and individuals as social beings require social healing in the form of trust-building in addition to whatever individual interventions are available.

The evidence on social inequalities reminds us that the stressors of life survival are generally highest among those with the lowest coping resources in terms of economic, social, or cultural capital. When inequalities are highly structured by social class, ethnic group, or some other division, then the risk of community level violence is always raised, and although the breakdown of the social fabric may have implications for all sectors, the deepest, most negative impacts are felt among the most disadvantaged citizens. I also consider the impact of violence on individuals as expressed in post-traumatic stress disorder (PTSD), not the only mental health problem to emerge in the wake of conflict but a disorder that has attracted most criticism.

Conflict

Much of the literature on trust dwells on the mechanisms of integration – how to minimise friction and conflict within society and between citizens and institutions. For economists, understanding the dynamics and determinants of trust is regarded as crucial to the efficient planning and running of organisations. For government, questions of trust are central to minimise conflict between communities or between citizens and government for the 'national good'. Given the rapidly changing global economic landscape, and high levels of international instability, the need to understand trust, if anything, has become more relevant. However, it is reasonable to suggest that the concept of trust was never a dominating topic in the social sciences let alone the sociology of health.

Much political and philosophical debate has focused on the polarised conceptualisation of human beings as either essentially cooperative or competitive. Famously, Thomas Hobbes viewed the latter as strongly determining human behaviour and relationships. Human beings left to their own devices, naturally competitive and forever seeking advantage over one another, would take society into dark miserable conditions 'nasty, brutish and short, a war of all against all'. In such a world, the problem of distrust can only be resolved through the strong, disciplining govern-ance of an overarching authority. The ruler didn't have to be benign, although a desirable quality, they were simply required to manage their subjects in a reason-ably equitable way so that subjects were less inclined to pursue their avaricious and violent impulses to the cost of the whole society. While people and communi-ties may remain distrustful, their rights and relationships, economic, and otherwise are underwritten by the sovereign. Immediately noticeable here is the relationship between trust, power, and vulnerability, allowing us to think around some of the definitions and parameters of each. Thus, for some academics, power is regarded as a set of interactions in a relationship, whereby one party achieves their desired outcome over those of another or as Max Weber described it, the likelihood that 'one actor within a social relationship will be in a position to carry out his own will despite the resistance of other participants' (Weber, 1964, p. 28). In this sense, power implies coercion or force to achieve these ends rather than the presence or use of authority – the social acceptance or acquiescence that the actor has the 'right' to exercise decision-making and ensure actions. This again, takes us into questions of legitimacy in authority; the ability to opt out of consent to this or that author-ity's rules and demands or where a 'benign' authority appears to have superficial consent and masks an ever-present threat of force. For example, as discussed in late sections, the legitimisation of diagnostic labelling by psychiatry and the ability determine coercive treatment for the individual, come to mind.

Routinisation and the avoidance of conflict

In the remaking of our worlds through routinisation and habit, ingrained and in-ternalised, these behaviours are employed, mostly unconsciously, in a web of ex-pectations through connected complex social systems whereby individuals and technology, for example, behave within an expected range of responses. Most of us ritually conform to quotidian practices related to dress, work, leisure, and family life that may appear stultifying but are comforting in that the absence of deviation or change reduces anxiety and stress. It is in this space that we touch upon argu-ably the most central of all sociological preoccupations – the maintenance of order when normative behaviours break down. The trust that emerges from expectations and predictability is a dimension of an accepted social script that allows families and communities to function smoothly. Goffman (1991) following on from his work on psychiatric patients within hospital institutions elaborated on the unwrit-ten rules and roles of individuals as social beings. Social norms are noted as a guide for action which are reinforced by various sanctions and rewards for infringements or maintenance, respectively. Mostly, people 'behave conventionally', engaging easily with others in a manner that is expected of them. If one was asked to de-scribe and justify these rules, the responses may well sound unintelligible or pecu-liar. It is when these expectations are breached, only then are the conventions and rules made visible. Garfinkle's (1967) breaching experiments or demonstrations in which the everyday conventions of speech or behaviours were challenged, revealed something about the disruption to composure and relationships. For example, in what should have been a usual greeting conversation between friends, a person (the experimenter) continually asked for clarification of commonly understood and quite uncontentious queries on general wellbeing; 'How are things?' might well be responded to by 'what do you mean – what things?'. In another experiment, students were instructed to behave at home as though they were lodgers – detached and polite. The students reported that other family members reacted with bewilderment and anger, and regarded the student as mean, nasty, and impolite. In these situations, it is the disruption of routinisation itself that provokes distress among other family and community members, the comfort and sense of security that the shared symbolic boundaries give to their interrelationships and interactions.

Distrust is recognised as both a determinant and an outcome of social conflict and violence, both of which can differ considerably in their expression, quality, and duration. As such, both run into difficulties of definition. For our purpose, we can simplify both to mean behaviours that constitute harmful disruption to social relations. From a Durkheimian perspective, the social provides a level of conditioning which supresses but doesn't eradicate the individual's instinctual or sometimes amoral impulses towards violence. An additional complication to the understanding of violence and conflict is the need for contextualising its expression and experience within specific socio-cultural frameworks. Thus, violence or the threat of violence cannot be explored as being ideal-typical, as possessing an inherent quality or character. Again, recalling Margaret Douglas on the issue of 'dirt as only matter out of place' (2002), acceptable conduct in one place and time, might be regarded as frightening and repugnant elsewhere; boxing and bullfighting come to mind. Caning and slapping schoolchildren are now outlawed in most Western societies but were once commonplace and may still be regarded as the moral prerogative of adults in some societies. Or similarly, social norms regarding the application of violent force in the control of people considered to be non-human or less than human.

Rapport and Overing (2007, p. 419) suggest that a more useful perspective on violence is to explore violence as 'a deliberate negation of formal routine and a refusal to enter into relations of mutual expectability through the perpetration of "disorderly" and unoriented behaviours'. Thus, in a bleakly neo-Hobbesian assessment, social structures are upheld by diverse people with varied and often incompatible needs only so far as they tacitly agree to mutually accommodate the other (or at least, not impede) in their activities. Accepting that all individuals are inherently violent, it is the relational routinisation or expectability that is the key factor in maintenance of order described by Rapport and Overing as 'democratic violence'. As long as behaviour is predictable (and thus, meaningful), the relationship can be maintained. Alternatively, 'nihilistic violence' is behaviour experienced by the other as meaningless and unpredictable, the violation of 'practicable norms of exchange' (Rapport & Overing, 2007, p. 421). The breakdown of norms of exchange and mutual expectations and which result in conflict, happen at both the macro- and the micro-levels, between nation states and between within communities, friendships, and marriages.

On the causal pathway to breakdown, mistrust is accompanied by other factors such as social inequalities and injustice, perceived or actual, and anxiety. The lack of trust in conflict settings may not force the cogs of social commerce and exchange to a grinding halt but generally, efficiency and wellbeing are denigrated. Conflicts, while depressingly similar in their destruction, injury, and loss of life, are dissimilar in terms of the geographical proximity and familiarity of the embroiled communities and populations. Like the 'thin' and 'thick' forms of trust, the depth of relationship and social connection matters considerably to the experience of betrayal and the impact of this on the mental health and recovery of communities and individuals.

Inequality, structural violence, and trust

Inequalities, either as perceived, relative, or absolute, provoke a dynamic of mistrust in which one group that owns or has access to some desirable goods or services, for example, seeks to defend its use from others. In this way, mistrust is thoroughly symbolised and projected through behaviours, whether through withdrawal or avoidance of stereotyped neighbourhoods and people or in the form of carrying weapons or living in gated communities and hiring security guards. These symbolic manifestations of mistrust, therefore, are both actively cause and consequence. Whether the challenges to inequality are regarded as the politics of envy, as commonly presented by conservative commentators, or as matter of social injustice, they are damaging to trust, health, and social cohesion, nevertheless (Merton, 1968).

Other evidence informs us that societies with higher levels of income inequality tend to be less trusting on average, a pattern also found in the relationship between income inequality and levels of happiness and anxiety (Van de Werfhorst & Salverda, 2012). In the United States, studies report between 50% and 75% of the variance in homicide rates and violent crime involving firearms is explained by high income inequality (Choe, 2008; Kennedy et al., 1998). International evidence indicates comparing different national statistics shows that income inequality is consistently associated with various crimes including homicide (van Wilsem, 2004). One study (Elgar & Aitken, 2010) which explored the relationship between income inequality and homicide rates across 33 countries noted that income inequality was implicated in significant international differences with income inequality accounting for nearly most of the variance in homicide rates controlling for per capita income differences. The Scandinavian countries and Japan all had relatively low inequality and homicide, alongside high levels of trust.

Whereas the 'hard-wired' nature of personality may be the least mutable to change, long-term population-based approaches to trust-building may be the most effective in increasing the wellbeing of citizens and reducing the prevalence of psychiatric disorders. Accordingly, there is much that society can do to build ambient trust and ameliorate the miseries created by mistrust, including conflict in the family and violence in society. Regardless of whether poor health and social outcomes are determined by psychosocial factors or more straightforwardly by poverty, it is hard to ignore the evidence that economic and other inequalities, the asymmetry of power, and the sense of injustice that these provoke are central explanatory factors to much human conflict.

Rothstein and Uslaner (2005) suggest that particularised trust reflects the shared bonds that cut across potential social divisions and communities (e.g. ethnic, religious, and class), conceptually similar to the notion of 'bridging' social capital. This is contrasted with particularised trust which is directed inwards towards one's own group. While increasing social pluralisation, the cross-pollination of ideas and the fluidity of sexual and gender identities may have dimmed the visibility of boundaries once heavily demarcated, most people remain geographically fixed within visible and intersecting communities of ethnicity and class. Social capital theory, at its conceptually thinnest, implies that the problems emerging from weak social cohesion may be located in the deficiencies of communities themselves, and policy-makers have happily picked up on this version of victim-blaming. Thus, the policy responses of many Western governments have been overly focussed on migration and ethnic diversity rather than producing an overarching and sustained approach to tackling the socio-economic processes related to the erosion and repairing of community connectedness and cohesion.[1]

Many of the countries that are high in particularised trust and low in generalised trust are recognisable by conspicuous inequalities out of which high rates of conflict, crime, and morbidity become more likely than countries in which these trust configurations are reversed. The perceived (or actual) threats posed by a toxic mixture of need and envy contribute to a vicious, self-perpetuating cycle of anxiety, mistrust, and conflict. The spread of highly policed segregated *gated communities* in the midst of poverty are a palpable reminder of the high cost of inequality and division. There is a need therefore for policy solutions that allow for more equitable redistribution of resources and opportunities that can assist in generating as much generalised trust as possible, while at the same time recognising that not all governments act in the best interest of all citizens and that in many instances, there is room for a healthy, informed mistrust.

Post-traumatic stress disorder (PTSD) and trust

Acting in the world with trust is largely done unconsciously, behaving with an internalised knowledge requiring no premeditation, otherwise much of our actions, even the mundane ones, would grind to almost paralysis. Moreover, much of what we have learned in childhood about the environment is experienced bodily rather than taught. As Camus suggests in *The Myth of Sisyphus* (2005), 'The body's judgement is as good as the mind's and the body shrinks from annihilation. We get into the habit of living before we get into the habit of thinking'. However, as we also learn that our environment and the objects within are not fixed; our knowledge of and responses to our worlds are generally contextual and contingent and may require adjustment in the light of other factors and change. The individual's navigation of the social world, although unconscious, is tested continually, absorbing and recalibrating. Humans tend to refine their capacity for avoiding suffering or improving effectiveness and survival. However, what happens when the individual's physical, mental, or moral integrity is violated?

Although exposed to violence or the trauma associated with conflict can experience multiple mental and physical disorders, the most commonly researched and reported in the psychiatric literature is PTSD (de Jong et al., 2001) with an estimated lifetime prevalence between 15% and 24% in Western societies. Over the past several decades, much of the research on PTSD relates to Vietnam War veterans but has since expanded to examine the consequences of natural disasters, physical and sexual violence, and childhood adversities in epidemiologic samples across various national settings.[2] There are various associated symptoms associated with PTSD which arise after the traumatic event(s) occurred. These include recurrent, intrusive memories of the event, distressing trauma-related dreams, dissociative reactions (e.g. flashbacks), intense or prolonged psychological distress, or physiological reactions at exposure to internal or external cues that symbolise or resemble an aspect of the traumatic event(s). Additionally, there may be persistent avoidance of distressing memories, thoughts, or feelings about the traumatic event(s) and marked change in arousal and reactivity, hypervigilance, irritability, and sleep disturbance. The person's symptoms may be accompanied by *depersonalisation*, a persistent of recurring sense of detachment from one's body or mind – or in a dream (Träum is German for dream), and *derealisation*, a sense of unreality in which the world is experienced as unreal or again, dreamlike.

An international expert on PTSD, Bessel Van Der Kolk (2014) noted a common response to trauma is an attempt by the individual to eradicate the very memory of the event, often unconsciously distancing oneself from the sense of shame, terror, or humiliation that often accompany such events, bearing in mind too that PTSD may be experienced by perpetrators as well as victims of traumatic events. The individual may employ various coping strategies, sometimes including alcohol or drug use but all requiring a considerable level of energy aimed at memory suppression, but in the absence of treatment attempts at managing the trauma, achieve only mental and physical exhaustion in the individual and those close to them. The attempts to suppress the unwanted memory/memories attached to the traumatic event may instead only serve to activate brain and body flooded by stress hormones to a 'present danger' from which the individual cannot escape. The emotional and physiological responses to PTSD can produce aggressive and destructive behaviour.

The neuroscientific evidence suggests that the reactions ensuing from traumatic events are not the product of flawed, difficult individuals, but rather they result from physical reconstructions in the brain. The shattering of assumptive worlds wrought by trauma applies to the individual's inner and outer worlds. The trust that life goes on as before is brought to a halt and this includes one's faith in a predictable self and the relationship with others and the environment. A diagnosis of PTSD and the symptoms commonly associated with it, generally fail to do justice to the phenomenological experiences in the lifeworld of the sufferer – the loss or threat of loss of control over emotions, feelings of entrapment, constant anxiety that lack a present object or cause. The world of the PTSD patient is rendered untrustworthy. More recently, the concept of complex PTSD has emerged defined as the consequence of a severe or protracted and repeated traumatisation leading to the disintegration of previously held values and views of the world, which then becomes untrustworthy and provoke transformations in personality, beliefs, and the distrust of people (Herman, 1992).

While the effects of war on combatants have been extensively examined, the medical literature of trauma among civilians has largely focussed on clinic-based populations of refugees (Summerfield, 2000). Particular diagnoses provide an indication, at least, for a particular treatment. The universal application of PTSD and consequent treatment implications have been challenged strongly by medical anthropologists and social psychologists (Bracken et al., 1995; Kleinman, 1981). However, while criticisms of PTSD as a Western social construct are valid, the collectivist-individualist dichotomy is somewhat overdone. The notion that Western societies are individualist and entirely lacking in collectivist cultural norms and behaviours doesn't hold nor is it credible to say, conversely, that people living in collectivist societies are incapable of feeling and acting on a sense of self. Individualist and collectivist personas are activated and reinforced for different reasons in different contexts. If we consider recent socio-political context of violence in some Western societies where the pull of communal, sectarian bonds are powerful and where an almost primal emotional loyalty to a mythical history of ancestral sacrifice runs deep, the individualist conception of values and motivations is less than convincing. Northern Ireland and the Balkans are two such recent examples. The most obvious concern is to understand the blend of engagement that is most helpful to people whose lives have been injured by conflict.

However, as noted earlier, the concept of PTSD and its universal applicability is highly contested. Making the point that all mental health diagnoses and psychological states are social constructs, Summerfield argues that PTSD is not a fixed entity across cultures nor even intra-culturally. What were once considered challenging occurrences, regarded as a test of character, are now psychiatric disorders requiring treatment (Summerfield, 2001). A rather contentious view holds that PTSD is about the only psychiatric disorder that is readily acceptable to a many people, implying that it carries little stigma because (a) the sufferer did not have a genetic predisposition to the illness, (b) the diagnosis brings benefits, and (c) it carries an exculpatory relief. In an echo of Parsons' (1951) sick role concept, once applied, PTSD provided the 'sufferer', services and society with a sanctioned illness, and an explanation for what would otherwise be deemed as weakness or 'bad' conduct. For those people seeking asylum, the state's response often depends on the ability to show 'objective' signs of suffering. For those whose scarring is more psychological than physical, the need to 'prove' the presence of PTSD through the loss of family and/or the witnessing of atrocious acts may be crucial to the success of asylum application (Eisenbruch, 1991; Richman, 1998; Sack et al., 1995). In such circumstances, notwithstanding the possibility that PTSD symptoms may not emerge for some years, it can be expected that refugees, or at least well-tutored refugees, are obliged to demonstrate all the convincing criteria of such problems underpinned by a convincingly coherent narrative. However, the philosopher and social theorist Slavoj Zizek makes the ironic point that the delivery of a coherent narrative following trauma is, of itself, incomprehensible: 'The very factual deficiencies of the traumatised subject's report on her experiences bear witness to the truthfulness of her report, since they signal that the reported content "contaminated" the manner of reporting it' (Zizek, 2008, p. 3).

For consideration then too is the extent to which different individuals resist or seek victim status. While there are financial or material gains attached to victim status, it is then likely that the attainment of victimhood will be positively correlated to social deprivation. Of course, the relatively deprived communities will suffer disproportionately in the course of conflict. The 'authentication' of PTSD opens the gateway to services and compensation; not just treatment for emotional and psychological problems but also the attainment of disability allowances and freedom from employment-seeking:

Thus, the politics of reparation, testimony and proof, demonstrate three practical ways in which trauma is applied to the field of action. In each of these three cases the focus is less on exacting empathy (although this intention may be present) or of representing oneself as a patient (although the expectation of treatment may be present) than on simply claiming one's rights. Thus, while trauma emerges in a context of an ethos of compassion that is characteristic of our era it is also a tool used in a demand for justice.

(Fassin & Rechtman, 2009, p. 279)

Moreover, the apparent marginal benefit is always relative to the possible alternatives that the individual can pursue or at least, perceives to be available and accessible. For example, an individual with low educational attainment in a family milieu of welfare dependency is likely to calculate the risks and rewards of sickness benefit very differently to a middle-class university graduate. Bourdieu's concept of *habitus* is helpful in suggesting that the cultural capital available to different groups will predispose individuals to different attitudes and courses of action. Thus, individuals desire and accommodate things that are familiar and available for them and disinclined to trust things which appear unfamiliar and of uncertain value (Bourdieu, 1977). Consequently, in working class and disadvantaged communities where welfare acceptance and dependency are generally and generationally entrenched, compensation is relatively more valued and more likely to be pursued. People from middle-class communities may be more inclined to view compensation as charity or welfare and less likely to engage with processes considered stigmatising in which some form of injury, often mental, has to be demonstrated to a panel of 'experts'. Conversely, civil servants and others in charge of the process have a 'built-in' mistrust of people who seek compensation, regarding them as part of a welfare culture and their claims of injury as inauthentic.

Community trauma and trust

The building of community trust is somewhat more complex and therefore challenging to achieve than overcoming individual trauma. Moreover, the latter may be impossible to fully achieve without the former. Thus, it is important to acknowledge that the impacts of conflict and trauma are widespread and deep with a collateral damage that creates waves and ripples through family life and across generations, a disruption of family milieu vacillating between silence and anger, filtering through into domestic injury, depressed spouses, and anxious children who vicariously absorb the damage. Thus, conflict is transferred from one 'battlefield' to the domestic and the personal, often rupturing the safety and security of families, commonly into future generations. Research on holocaust survivors and children of people impacted by conflict indicates that there may be an intergenerational effect associated with exposure to extensive or long-term trauma (Solomon et al., 1988). A growing body of theory and empirical research is uncovering the relationships between shame, trauma, and violence (Gilligan, 2000). Thus, Gilligan has argued persuasively from his therapeutic work with violent offenders in the US penal system and drawing on psychological and social anthropological theories of violence that the origins of much violence can be located in actual or perceived threats to the self and the compendium of negative emotional responses that follow – a sense of shame, devaluation, humiliation, and loss of honour (Gilligan, 2001, pp. 31–37; Scheff & Retzinger, 1991).[3] As explored in other parts of this book, childhood experiences of abuse and humiliation contribute to and perpetuate cycles of violence; however, that violence is expressed. Importantly, in the way that Arendt suggests, violence rather than peace is the continuum in human history. Accordingly, as she points out, the end of the Second World War in 1945 did not herald peace but in the birth of the so-called 'cold war' and the sporadic emergence of other wars globally.

Rebuilding trust in post-conflict societies

How trauma in post-conflict societies is conceptualised and managed is contentious in terms of government policy and service provision for people considered as victims. For example, generally discussed as 'the troubles' or the 'Northern Irish conflict' has had widespread and damaging impacts across the island of Ireland and Great Britain. To some extent, the statistics on the conflict in places such as Northern Ireland[4] only reflect the measurable impacts of the conflict – injuries and deaths; harder to comprehend and illustrate are the intangible, seemingly immeasurable consequences of prolonged violence and threat. At the outer circles of conflict impact, everybody was changed and affected to some degree. Whatever trust existed between communities prior to the conflict's outbreak rapidly dissolved. City and town centres were left deserted at nighttime as people retreated to the relative safety of heavily fortified venues in their own locales. In addition, intra-communal violence, often so-called 'punishment beatings', was a prevalent feature of community life.

Out of the fear of sectarian atrocities and the cycle of retaliation emerged a dysregulation of social behaviour and attitudes that, at least outwardly, became normalised and acceptable. Hypervigilance with regard to threat of violence and constant self-protection measures became a part of everyday life. The intangible impacts of conflict include the lost opportunities in terms of education and employment for many of those caught up in violence and the increasing acceptability of violence itself within the community and the family. For many others too, the conflict, interlinked with the high levels of unemployment, provoked departure and exile.

As part of its 'peace process', the needs of victims and survivors in which the provision of psychological therapies is a major policy issue. However, as in other conflict settings, and here one can include disadvantaged urban areas where violence is commonplace, the focus on individual suffering and treatment, while may also be of limited value in the long-run, divisive and problematic. Thus, the criteria used to define and label 'victims' are morally and politically infused. In this context, the assignment of 'trauma' status, leading to treatment or compensation, is assigned a legitimising and rationing significance. In civil conflicts, individuals deemed to be participants are commonly excluded as undeserving treatment, with the potential of undermining social cohesion provoking a return to violent behaviour. This may be a failure to acknowledge the determinants of social conflict, namely inequalities and distrust. Moreover, targeted psychological treatment provided to individuals may be useful but of limited benefit to many victims and unacceptable to others.

Targeted psychological interventions overshadow the collateral and more diffuse impacts of civil conflict that have become, over several generations, enmeshed with problems that pre-existed the conflict and likely intensified in consequence. Here we consider problems of social exclusion and family dysregulation, addictions, and mental illness. Seldom acknowledged, peace often brings increased wealth and status for some social strata, professional groups, and entrepreneurs, leading to produce further alienation and social tensions. Thus, such a scenario exists in post-apartheid South Africa whereby the expected socio-economic benefits of political 'settlement' in the new 'rainbow nation' never quite trickled down to people at the lower echelons (Struwig et al., 2011). To achieve a flourishing post-conflict society, there is a need to focus resources and energies on mental health initiatives that simultaneously build resilience at the personal and the communal levels. The vision must include trust-building and a transformation from individual and community 'victimhood' to empowered survivorship.

Conflict and mental illness

The return to 'normality' for many is a surrender of community status and power. As the rationale for violent conflict diminishes, there tends to be an increase in rates of substance abuse, relationship breakdown, domestic violence, and mood disorders.[5] While psycho-social problems are high in the general population, they are higher again among ex-combatants (Anckermann et al., 2005; Jarman, 2004). For example, in an epidemiological study of almost 5,000 people in Somaliland, 20% of families, more than a decade post-conflict, were caring for one or more family members, predominantly ex-combatants, who had severe mental problems and comorbidly abusing khat, an indigenous narcotic. These ex-fighters were twice as likely to experience mental illness than civilian survivors (Odenwald et al., 2005). There is evidence that psychiatric disorders emerge or become known to service many years post-conflict (Utzon-Frank et al., 2014). To anyone caught up in neighbourhoods where violence and the threat of violence are prevalent but the opportunities for escape are limited, an accommodation of threat and anxiety may permit survival and continuity in the present but which have to be 'paid for' at some later point.

Rebuilding trust

In tightly knit communities where violence is condensed and more acutely psychologically felt, PTSD or at least the dominant characteristics of trauma events (e.g. hypervigilance, insomnia, and avoidance) are commonly experienced. If a significant proportion of any population experience trauma symptoms and other conflict-related psychiatric disorders, what then should be done in order to address such problems? It seems an obvious point to make that entrenched social problems and their psychological correlates are reproduced over generations in what is clearly a systemic problem rather than simply a problem of individual pathology. However, while it is generally assumed that the presence of PTSD symptoms is determined by direct exposure to war-related violence, recent evidence suggests that 'structural' adversities and stressors may have greater predictive power than war exposure (Miller & Rasmussen, 2010). Moreover, while the importance of building social capital in repairing the psychological and social damage wrought by conflict is often stated, how this is operationalised is poorly understood. Social capital elements such as trust and reciprocity make social capital as a construct intuitively 'correct' but only within a 'bonding' social capital that also excludes the 'outsider'. Thus, in a sectarianised environment bonding social capital may only bolster division, simultaneously strengthening a trust that is communally limited and introspective, while denying the possibility of an expansive, society-wide trust.[6]

There is a strong case that social ecology or environmental approaches should be the first line of provision because without these in place, individualised therapies are greatly reduced in their effectiveness. Kaethe Weingarten, a Harvard-based clinical psychologist, has worked with survivors of conflict and trauma and has written extensively on the concept of 'witnessing' which emphasises the collateral damage done by acts of violence and hurt, widening the breadth of effect beyond those in the immediate nexus (victim-perpetrator).

This widening of effect is important in more fully considering how trauma, suffering, and healing are considered at the individual and the social levels. Thus, Martın-Baro (1990) indicates that conflict-related post-traumatic reactions are incomprehensible when they are solely at the individual level because such reactions are embedded in a historical, social contexts. Interventions aimed at alleviating suffering must address the social fabric of the community because social relationships and conditions can either exacerbate or attenuate the individual's experience of suffering or traumatic stress. The depth of the social permeation of suffering suggests that the reconstruction of the social fabric is an inescapable element of individual healing and flourishing (Anckermann et al., 2005). Psychosocial approaches emphasise the importance of the individual's environment in exacerbating or alleviating psychological distress. Thus, attention is given to supportive family and community networks, enhancing community-based resources, and alleviating or removing exposure to harmful daily stressors. As previously argued, the absence of trust is a space often saturated with negative emotions and behaviours such as insecurity, anxiety, and hypervigilance – not exactly the conditions in which well-being can thrive.

Post-conflict policies may be a useful context in which to consider the contested nature of trauma and victimhood and the potential advantage offered by preventative and community approaches. The dysregulation within post-conflict means that that the criteria and defining of victims and survivors are often too restrictive, potentially invalidating the suffering (indirect, hidden, or not considered) of many people who have become the collateral victims of conflict sequelae.

Peace settlements seldom make allowance for transitional justice programmes beyond the investigation of highly contentious incidents. Instead, the parties to such agreements concentrate on developing frameworks within which the violence of the past could be acknowledged impartially and the needs of individuals impacted by conflict managed as far as possible. However, in defining 'victims' and 'survivors', the conflict and its impacts are reduced to discrete incidents, a direct line between cause and effect. Significantly, the definition excludes the concept of accumulative and/or indirect suffering. While limited resources demand rationing, they also inevitably result in 'winners and losers' and prologued feelings of injustice. Thus, the membership of this 'group' is highly contested. First, it is often politically unfeasible to give universal recognition to the traumatising effects of violence. There is a political inability to offer parity between citizens and combatants, sustaining a view that dichotomises these categories and rejecting the possibility of dual-membership. Such a position also denies a common humanity, which neutralises moral categories of innocence and guilt? (See Fassin & Rechtman for a discussion on US troops in Vietnam; 2009, pp. 91–93.) Moreover, such dichotomies may only serve to foster resentment and future violent conflict on the basis of deserving and non-deserving individuals through the assignment of innocence and blame and hierarchies of suffering. Importantly, the degree of suffering or impact on victims of violence is of immense significance as a mechanism for compensation and the provision of appropriate health and social services. Is it possible to differentiate and thus adjudicate on a moral basis the provision of goods and services according to an individual's relationship and/or contribution to civil conflict?

Conflicts, which are ultimately resolved through one side overcoming the other, tend not to face the dilemma of victim-perpetrator defining. Post-conflict initiatives such as truth recovery commissions are often partial and impartial, reflecting the political will of the dominant group. Thus, victor-vanquished demarcations generally also delineate innocence and guilt. However, in post-conflict societies where violent conflict is ended, albeit partially, through negotiation, categories of innocence and guilt require a strong degree of 'bracketing out', a wilful avoidance of apportioning blame. To apportion blame in the context of conflict, however, is also to assign levels of trust and trustworthiness.

The focus on individual trauma which secures treatment to the relative neglect of a wider social and community dysfunction is of questionable merit. Thus, the term 'victim' is weighted with meaning and significance, altering the perception and the type of engagement of others. For the person thus labelled, there is an alteration from autonomous agent to passive 'object' whose suffering can be treated medically (and/or alleviated through financial compensation). Importantly, the acceptance of the label 'victim' as a contractual arrangement has worrying implications for the relationship between the state and the individual, sanctioning a type of behaviour that is commensurate with the label, encouraging illness behaviour and a de facto creation of 'victimhood'.[7] Trust in this context is double-edged. Clinically, a diagnosis of PTSD is an authentication of an account of mentally injurious event(s); the person's suffering is to be trusted. Conversely, a diagnosis of PTSD also indicates a removal of trust in the person's ability to function capably.

Fassin and Rechtman (2009) argue, we cannot know how 'victims' view themselves

> we know nothing of their subjectivity – or interiority – as victims. They adopt the only persona that allows them to be heard – that of victim. In doing so they tell us less about what they are than the moral economies of our era in which they find their place. Victims may have to assume the status without agreeing to the status or condoning the process by which they achieve it.[8] Taking great care not to examine the truthfulness of trauma claims, in pushing this perspective we are challenged to examine the specificities of place and time and what our management of victims say about social relations and political situations. The social construction of trauma (as a means of illuminating and describing the wounds of the past) is to selectively choose those deemed to be victims and, despite its assumed universality, produces disparities with regards to whom will benefit from treatment.[9]
>
> (Fassin & Rechtman, 2009, p. 282)

They also make the case that cultural, social, and ontological proximity are significant in the assessment of trauma as does an evaluation of the trustworthiness about the cause and validity of the suffering, and in doing so, initiates a hierarchy of legitimacy among victims. Trauma is therefore less of a psychological state or clinical reality but increasingly, a moral and political judgement.

Johan Galtung's (1969) dual perspective on violence and peace argued that the establishment of peace is not simply the absence of violence.[10] Thus, he rejects the usual narrow concept of violence as actions intentionally perpetrated by one person on another's body preferring a much wider conceptualisation in which 'violence is present when human beings are being influenced so that their actual somatic and mental realizations are below their potential realizations'. If peace is simply defined as the negation of somatic violence, the bar is set too low, giving permission to a myriad of unacceptable actions that can be accommodated within a peaceful state. Thus conceptualised, detention without trial, intimidation, and psychological torture are all permitted. Violence, he argues, is not just the perpetration of bodily or mental harm, though these are important, but rather the difference between people's potential for health and development and their actual realisation of this potential. Thus, public health approaches aimed at restoring inter-community trust, equality, and security, supplemented by individual therapies where appropriate, may offer best hope for lasting wellbeing.

Notes

1 Additionally, academic interest in community cohesion has been hampered by low interdisciplinarity, a highly localised focus, and generally lacking in the longer-term observation of macro and micro determinants of trust and cohesion. Moreover, there is a need to obtain a better understanding of social cohesion as differently experienced and acknowledged by diverse stakeholders (Fonseca et al., 2019).

2 The Diagnostic and Statistical Manual of Mental Disorders (DSM-5 Diagnostic Criteria for PTSD) requires that the person had 'Exposure to actual or threatened death, serious injury, or sexual violence in one (or more) of the following ways (1) Directly experiencing the traumatic event(s); (2) Witnessing, in person, the event(s) as it occurred to others; (3) Learning that the traumatic event(s) occurred to a close family member or close friend. In cases of actual or threatened death of a family member or friend, the event(s) must have been violent or accidental; (4) Experiencing repeated or extreme exposure to aversive details of the traumatic event(s) (e.g., first responders collecting human remains; police officers repeatedly exposed to details of child abuse). **Note:** Criterion A4 does not apply to exposure through electronic media, television, movies, or pictures, unless this exposure is work related'.

3 In the many conflict situations, this linkage may be detected. Arguably, the origins of the Second World War are acknowledged to result from a profound sense of German national dishonour and humiliation provoked by the allied powers.

4 How should the scale of the conflict be depicted or quantified? Who do we define as having suffered or witnessed violence? Perhaps the simplest way would be to describe the statistics of loss and destruction. Thus, in Northern Ireland between 1969 and 2001, 3,523 people were killed as a result of the conflict most of whom (53%) were civilians (Eames & Bradley, 2009) rather than those people identified in some way as combatants (i.e. members of the British army, Loyalist, or Republican paramilitary groups).

The scale of the conflict can be further apprehended when we also include in the statistics, the lives damaged of approximately 47,000 people who were injured and disabled through bombing ($N = 16,200$) and shooting incidents ($N = 37,000$). However, we can also widen the circles of impact to include the disruption to normal communal life by 22,500 armed robberies and 2,200 arson attacks. Moreover, families and communities faced upheaval in the context of almost 20,000 individuals imprisoned for scheduled offences and many others detained without trial.

5   McDonald (2007), a consultant psychiatrist working in Belfast throughout the troubles, observed that people who were active in conflict tend to cope well with the emotional consequences of what has been done to them and what they have done to others but only just as long as their actions can be justified towards a greater end, that is, while their actions and suffering have meaning. For many ex-combatants, participation in conflict provides a tenuous and temporary platform for social status generally absent in unequal societies.

6   The so-called 'peace-walls' in Northern Ireland, increasing in number since the Good Friday Agreement, embody the paradox of social capital in the midst of fear and distrust.

7   Labelling theory concerns the self-identity and behaviour individuals that may be determined by the labels or terms employed to describe or categorise them. It is often linked to the notion of a self-fulfilling prophecy.

8   Many people will not readily self-label as victim but if its acceptance is the only portal to other material and psychological/emotional benefits, at least in the short term, there is certainly an incentive to do so. However, those people who reject the label, while nevertheless having unexpressed needs, are excluded from obtaining appropriate help. If needs are determined on the basis of self-identified victim status, it is likely that the distribution of services will be inequitable and not commensurate with level of need.

9   The authors note that treatment for PTSD is not readily provided in Rwanda and other African countries.

10 Galtung's broad conceptualisation of peace has three basic principles '1. That the term "peace" shall be used for social goals at least verbally agreed to by many, if not necessarily by most. 2. These social goals may be complex and difficult, but not impossible, to attain. 3. The statement peace is absence of violence shall be retained as valid'. In providing as broad a definition as possible, he provides an 'orientation in favor of peace compatible with a number of ideologies outlining other aspects of social orders'. His conceptualisation of violence is obliged to be commensurate with his understanding of peace.

References

Anckermann, S., Dominguez, M., Soto, N., Kjaerulf, F., Berliner, P., & Mikkelsen, E. N. (2005). Psycho-social support to large numbers of traumatized people in post-conflict societies: An approach to community development in Guatemala. *Journal of Community & Applied Social Psychology, 15*, 136–152.

Arendt, H. (1970). *On violence*. Harcourt.

Berger, P., & Luckman, T. (1966). *The social construction of reality*. Doubleday.

Bourdieu, P. (1977). *Outline of a theory of practice*. Cambridge University Press.

Bracken, P. J., Gillera, J. E., & Summmerfield, D. (1995). Psychological responses to war and atrocity: The limitations of current concepts. *Social Science and Medicine, 40*(8), 1073–1082.

Camus, A. (2005). *The myth of Sisyphus*. Penguin.

Choe, J. (2008). Income inequality and crime in the United States. *Economics Letters, 101*(1), 31–33.

de Jong, J. T. V. M., Komproe, I. H., Van Ommeren, M., El Masri, M., Araya, M., Khaled, N., van de Put, W., & Somasundaram, D. (2001). Lifetime events and posttraumatic stress disorder in 4 postconflict settings. *JAMA, 286*(5), 555–562. https://doi.org/10.1001/jama.286.5.555

Douglas, M. (2002). *Purity and danger*. Routledge. (1966).

Durkheim, E. (1897). *Suicide*. The Free Press reprint 1997.

Eames, R., & Bradley, D. (2009). *Report of the consultative group on the past*. https://cain.ulster.ac.uk/victims/docs/consultative_group/cgp_230109_report.pdf

Eisenbruch, M. (1991). From post-traumatic stress disorder to cultural bereavement: Diagnosis of Southeast Asian refugees. *Social Science & Medicine, 33*(6), 673–680.

Elgar, F. J., & Aitken, N. (2010). Income inequality, trust and homicide in 33 countries. *European Journal of Public Health, 21*(2), 241–246. https://doi.org/10.1093/eurpub/ckq068

Fassin, D., & Rechtman, R. (2009). *The empire of trauma*. Princeton University Press.

Fonseca, X., Lukosch, S., & Brazier, F. (2019). Social cohesion revisited: A new definition and how to characterize it. *Innovation: The European Journal of Social Science Research, 32*(2), 231–253. https://doi.org/10.1080/13511610.2018.1497480

Galtung, J. (1969). Violence, peace, and peace research. *Journal of Peace Research, 6*(3), 167–191. https://doi.org/10.1177/002234336900600301

Garfinkel, H. (1967). *Studies in ethnomethodology*. Prentice-Hall.

Gilligan, J. (2000). *Violence: Reflections on our deadliest epidemic*. Jessica Kingsley.

Gilligan, J. (2001). *Preventing violence*. Thams Hudson.

Goffman, E. (1991). *Asylums: Essays on the social situation of mental patients and other inmates*. Penguin.

Herman, J. L. (1992). Complex PTSD: A syndrome in survivors of prolonged and repeated trauma. *Journal of Traumatic Stress, 5*(3), 377–391. https://doi.org/10.1002/jts.2490050305

Jarman, N. (2004). From war to peace, changing patterns of violence in Northern Ireland 1990–2003. *Terrorism and Political Violence, 16*(3), 420–438.

Kennedy, B. P., Kawachi, I., Prothrow-Stith, D., Lochner, K., & Gupta, V. (1998). Social capital, income inequality, and firearm violent crime. *Social Science & Medicine, 47*(1), 7–17.

Kleinman, A. (1981). *Patients and healers in the context of culture; An exploration of the borderland between anthropology, medicine and psychiatry*. University of California Press.

Krug, E. G., Dahlberg, L. L., Mercy, J. A., Zwi, A. B., & Lozano, R. (2002). *World report on violence and health*. Lancet. 2002 Oct 5;360(9339):1083–8. doi: 10.1016/S0140-6736(02)11133-0. PMID: 12384003.

Martın-Baro, I. (1990). La violencia politica y la guerra como causas del trauma psicosocial en El Salvador [The political violence and the war as causes of psychosocial trauma in El Salvador]. In I. Martın-Baro (Ed.), *Psicologı´a social de la guerra: Trauma y terapia. Social psychology of war: Trauma and therapy*. UCA Editores.

McDonald, G. (2007). Mental health consequences of long term conflict. *British Medical Journal, 334*, 1121–1122.

Merton, R. K. (1968). *Social theory and social structure*. Simon and Schuster.

Miller, K. E., & Rasmussen, A. (2010). War exposure, daily stressors, and mental health in conflict and post-conflict settings: bridging the divide between trauma-focused and psychosocial frameworks. *Social Science & Medicine, 70*(1), 7–16. https://doi.org/10.1016/j.socscimed.2009.09.029

Odenwald, M., Neuner, F., Schauer, M., Elbert, T., Catani, C., Lingenfelder, B., Hinkel, H., Häfner, H., & Rockstroh, B. (2005). Khat use as risk factor for psychotic disorders: A cross-sectional and case-control study in Somalia. *BMC Medicine, 3*, 5. https://doi.org/10.1186/1741-7015-3-5

Parsons, T. (1951). *The social system*. Free Press.

Rapport, N., & Overing, J. (2007). *Social and cultural anthropology: The key concepts.* Routledge.

Richman, N. (1998). Refugees and asylum seekers in the West. In P. Bracken & C. Petty (Eds.), *Rethinking the trauma of war* (pp. 170–186). Free Association Press.

Rothstein, B., & Uslaner, E. M. (2005). All for all: Equality, corruption, and social trust. *World Politics, 58*(1), 41–72. https://doi.org/10.1353/wp.2006.0022

Sack, W. H., Clarke, G., & Steely, J. (1995). Post-traumatic stress disorder across two generations of Cambodian refugees. *Journal of the American Academy of Child and Adolescent Psychiatry, 34,* 1160–1166.

Scheff, T., & Retzinger, S. (1991). *Emotions and violence: Shame and rage in destructive conflicts.* Lexington.

Simmel, G. (1955). *Conflict & the web of group affiliations.* The Free Press.

Solomon, Z., Kotler, M., & Mikulincer, M. (1988). Combat-related posttraumatic stress disorder among second-generation Holocaust survivors: Preliminary findings. *American Journal of Psychiatry, 145,* 865–868.

Struwig, J., Davids, Y. D., Roberts, B., Sithole, M., Tilley, V., Weir-Smith, G., & Mokhele, T. (2011). *Towards a social cohesion barometer for South Africa. Somerset West, South Africa.*

Summerfield, D. (2000). War and mental health: A brief overview. *British Medical Journal, 321,* 232–235.

Summerfield, D. (2001). The invention of post-traumatic stress disorder and the social usefulness of a psychiatric category. *British Medical Journal, 322*(7278), 95–98. https://doi.org/10.1136/bmj.322.7278.95

Utzon-Frank, N., Breinegaard, N., Bertelsen, M., Borritz, M., Eller, N. H., Nordentoft, M., Olesen, K., Rod, N. H., Rugulies, R., & Bonde, J. P. (2014). Occurrence of delayed-onset post-traumatic stress disorder: A systematic review and meta-analysis of prospective studies. *Scandinavian Journal of Work, Environment & Health, 40*(3), 215–229. https://doi.org/10.5271/sjweh.3420

Van de Werfhorst, H. G., & Salverda, W. (2012). Consequences of economic inequality: Introduction to a special issue. *Research in Social Stratification and Mobility, 30*(4), 377–387. https://doi.org/10.1016/j.rssm.2012.08.001

Van Der Kolk, B. (2014). *The body keeps the score: Mind, brain and body in the transformation of trauma.* Penguin.

van Wilsem, J. (2004). Criminal victimization in cross-national perspective: An analysis of rates of theft, violence and vandalism across 27 countries. *European Journal of Criminology, 1*(1), 89–109. https://doi.org/10.1177/1477370804038708

Weber, M. (1964). *The theory of social and economic organization.* The Free Press.

Zizek, S. (2008). *Violence.* Profile.

Chapter 4

Alienation and Trust

Berger and Luckman argue that beliefs about the nature and content of social reality emerges through social processes in which the internalisation of the 'socially objectivated world are *the same* processes that internalize the socially assigned identities' (Berger & Luckman, 1966, p. 16). Particularly important in the context of mental illness and how it comes to be created and defined by others, individuals appropriate the world through conversation and interaction with others, thus allowing the world and identity to 'remain real' but only inasmuch as the 'conversation' with others can be maintained. Moreover, Berger and Luckman emphasise that the process of socialisation is an on-going lifetime process which is inherently precarious: 'The difficulty of keeping a world going expresses itself psychologically in the difficulty of keeping this world subjectively plausible'. Moreover, if the maintenance of reality depends on ongoing dialogue with significant others, the disruption caused by illness, death, or migration, for example, "the world begins to totter, to lose its subjective reality. In other words, the subjective reality of the world hangs on the thread of these conversations. The only reason why most of us are unaware of this precariousness most of the time is grounded in the continuity of conversation with significant others".

Although Berger and Luckman focus on the maintenance of religious beliefs in society, the social construction of reality has wider significance. Without continued interaction with others, plausibility structures begin to crumble. Disconnection with other people with similar beliefs, or simply the loss of connection with others, leaves the individual as a 'cognitive alien'.

If humans are obliged to 'impose a meaningful order upon society' based on a 'social enterprise of ordering world construction', as Berger and Luckman (1966) suggest, 'the individual's separation from society exposes him or her to unbearable psychological pain created by a meaninglessness, a "nightmare *par excellence*" in which the individual is submerged in a world of disorder, senselessness and madness' (p. 22). With striking emphasis, they suggest that sanity is predicated on *being in* society in that this presence protects us from the terror of anomie. Thus, individuals may prefer to die than surrender to meaninglessness.

DOI: 10.4324/9781003326687-4

Suicide suggests the failure of conversations which may have offered alternative choices. In this chapter, I explore some of these lifetime 'conversations', particularly those that begin in childhood and provide a 'script' for living with trust or mistrust. Whether we approach the social world with either trust or mistrust, how we anticipate the intentions of others towards us depends to a considerable extent on our exposure to previous events and experiences, the cultural microcosm of family life, and more specifically on problems in the development of a relationship between child and parent. Thus, the individual's social skills and dispositions formed in childhood and by their early environment influence mental health and relationships. Importantly, the origins of loneliness and various mental health problems are associated with these early experiences. Mental disorders in themselves can be considered as a breakdown in self-trust as much as they are related to a rupture with reality. When the assessment of reality is uncertain, incoherent, or disputed, the ability to trust other people, systems, or the future is fraught.

Childhood adversity, attachment, and loss of trust

The accumulated evidence from major international studies suggests that approximately a third of individuals have been exposed to various types of childhood maltreatment which comprises any kind of abusive act (sexual, violence, or verbal) or neglect with consequent physical or emotional harm, potential for harm, or threat of harm to a child (CDC, 2008). For example, the child may have been exposed to interparental violence and parental substance use. The impact of childhood maltreatment, commonly referred to adverse childhood events (ACEs), is often severe and enduring with increased risks for a range of psychiatric disorders, including depression, anxiety, post-traumatic stress disorder (PTSD), personality disorders, and substance misuse (Hughes et al., 2017). Biomedical evidence highlights the impact of ACEs on neurological, hormonal, and immunological development, revealing increasing biomarkers for inflammation and shortened telomeres (Danese & McEwen, 2012) from which comes an increased risk of chronic and life-limiting physical conditions including cardiovascular disease and diabetes (Su et al., 2015). Cumulatively, those experience adversity in childhood have an increased risk of disease development due to differences in physiological development and engagement in health-damaging behaviours. Indeed, meta-analysis data indicates that people who experienced childhood adversity had a seven-fold risk of violence victimisation and an eight-fold risk for violence perpetration (Hughes et al., 2017).

The impacts of adversity are also transferred to the next generation. A recent study of almost 4,000 mothers of whom 44% had experienced childhood exposure to abuse or neglect and were more likely to have children with internalising problems of clinical significance, autism spectrum disorder, attention-deficit hyperactivity disorder (ADHD), and physical health comorbidities. The study also showed a dose–response relationship in that those with multiple adversities were more at risk of poor health outcomes (Moog et al., 2023).

The significance of child-parent bonding for life-long mental health and wellbeing has a 'taken for granted' understanding, not just within clinical academic circles but among health practitioners, policy-makers, and general public. It wasn't always this way. Until John Bowlby's observations about the impact of a disrupted maternal relationship among juvenile 'delinquents' and 'maladapted' children, social learning and psychoanalytic theory credited child-mother bonding for the pleasure received by the child on satiation of the hunger drive. While dealing with hunger is obviously important, animal observational studies indicated that infants can become attached to non-feeding parents. Some mechanism other than secondary learning must explain attachment. Child-parent observation studies from the 1950s and 1960s demonstrated the importance of proximity between parent and child as crucial to the roots and alleviation of distress. Briefly, all biologically-based attachment behaviours such as signalling (smiling and volatilising) to attract the parent's attention to the child's desire for interaction or aversive (crying) to attract the parent in order to diminish distress. Bowlby proposed an evolutionary explanation for attachment behaviour in which genetic selection favoured such behaviours because they boosted the chances of child-mother proximity, which consequently increased the probability of safety and thus, provided a survival advantage. However, Bowlby later downplayed the evolutionary behavioural adaptation in attachment in order to state its multiple benefits such as feeding, self-regulation, and social connectedness which all add to an evolutionary advantage (Cassidy, 2016, p. 5). Bowlby noted that a child's goal in attachment behaviour is not primarily the connection with the 'object' (i.e. the mother), but rather a state, a 'behavioural homeostasis' regulated by the desired distance from the mother. The child's distress is controlled through a level of contact with the mother, contingent on the level of activation in the attachment system.

Over time, the parent-child attachment experiences are internalised into what Bowlby described as internal working models (IWMs), essentially cognitive representations or models of caregiving experiences which in turn provide a template for later interpersonal behaviour and relationships with others. Thus, 'continual transactions with the world of persons and objects, the child constructs increasingly complex internal working models of that world and of the significant persons in it, including the self'. These models permit a degree of future planning and decision-making – autonomy, permissible actions in exploring, adventure and creativity, and so on. While attachment may hold the key to the infant's safety and survival, the secure base is only beneficial in the long-run if it permits exploratory behaviour, the opportunity to develop a healthy and productive engagement with the environment. The proximity and availability of an attachment figure can be sufficiently reassuring for the child to permit exploration. A dynamic equilibrium is created when the distance created by either the mother's or child's movement is monitored and when necessary, restored to mutual contentment. The development and testing of trust is at the core of this dynamic dialectical exchange between child and attachment figure; both independently, assessing the child's exploratory boundaries and the child evaluating the trustworthiness of parental intervention.

However, these internalised models of the world are not static, but rather adapt to the child's developing affective-cognitive knowledge whereby sense of self, others, and environment become increasingly sophisticated (Bretherton, 1985), accompanied by changes in attachment system behaviours. Over time, more nuanced attachment behaviour is observed in children as they become more skilled in assessing and anticipating the wishes and intentions of attachment figures. In so doing, they learn to calculate risk more accurately and cope with distress. Cassidy proposes the term 'caregiving system' to describe a set of specific parental behaviours which promote proximity and comfort when the parent senses that the child is in danger or distress, real or potential. Retrieval is the most obvious of these behaviours which include 'calling, reaching, restraining, following, soothing and rocking' (Cassidy, 2016, p. 10). Crucially for an understanding of how childhood attachment relates to trust, mental health, and help-seeking, we should begin to grasp how these internalised models impact on their apprehension of themselves and the world. The internalised working models are highly predicated on the responses of the attachment figure.

When parental responses are inconsistent, children show less trust in the environment, bringing more attention to the parent but accompanied by uncertainty that they will respond when required and demonstrated by an insistence on close proximity to the parent. Conversely, children who experience the parent as constantly unresponsive during episodes of distress are more likely to switch attention to the environment in an attempted suppression of growing negative emotions and the avoidance of parental insensitivity. Distrust in parental availability can produce avoidant or dismissing attachment (Cassidy, 2016). Where comforting responses to a child's distress are withheld, erratic, or contemptuous, for example, the child is more likely to develop a model of the parent as undependable, untrustworthy, or rejecting, but this is coterminous with a self-evaluation of being someone unworthy of love and comfort. Contrariwise, timely, loving, and reassuring responses from an attachment figure are consonant with a more benign self-evaluation. These dyadic constructions of self through the internalised working models help build the capacity for intergenerational transfer of helpful and unhelpful cognitions and behaviours. According to Bretherton, 'a child who trusts the parents to give needed emotional support will also learn the complementary parental role and be able to enact it later when he or she becomes a parent' (Bretherton, 1985).

Bretherton tells us that 'optimal ontogenetic adaptation of the attachment system occurs under circumstances in which major caregivers accept the child's needs' is implicit in Bowlby's and Ainsworth's work' in which the attachment system has a core bias arising from its evolutionary basis but sufficiently adaptive to various caregiver behaviours. However, somewhat problematically, there is no universal set of caregiving behaviours. They may differ considerably within and between cultures, provoking the possibility of attachment theory as restricted to Western culture. That is not to state that the concept of attachment behaviours has value only in Western societies, but rather caregiving styles in different cultural contexts require deeper exploration (Rothbaum et al., 2000).

The delicacy and plasticity of the brain has been acknowledged for some time. A considerable body of evidence from rodent, primate, and human research tells a consistent story about severe, recurrent stressors at critical developmental periods producing changes in multiple brain circuits and systems that have enduring, often permanent, neurobehavioral effects across the life course (Teicher et al., 2003). These effects increase the risk of developing depression, personality disorder, PTSD, and substance abuse. They are also associated with symptoms of ADHD (Teicher et al., 2002). Additionally, among individuals exposed to trauma, the neural capacities in coping with or regulating stress arousal levels are often seriously compromised (Frewen & Lanius, 2006). These early childhood experiences and their neurological sequelae may also lay the foundations for loneliness into adulthood.

The adverse events described earlier are always located in the context of power, commonly asymmetrical, and sometimes accompanied by violence – physical, psychological, or sexual. Even where children are not exposed to the structural violence of poverty, the potential for generalised trust is critically hampered. Childhood vulnerability and dependency means that the conditions for trust towards those in power are either irrelevant or unlikely to be present. As we shall explore, adverse events and experiences, and how individuals respond to them, will have considerable consequences for mental health over the life course. Importantly, while much of the literature on trust is occupied by discussions of its salience in the smooth running of life and relationships in different fields, in many situations or contexts, trust is surely not the sensible or logical response. In the presence of bad actors, familiarity with the 'other' is a strong motivation for mistrust.

When anxiety, or perhaps fear, arises as a result of an individual's uncertainty or ambivalence about or person (or institution) not directly responsible or connected to the original violation of trust, it is commonly regarded as neurotic behaviour or much more negatively, as a mental illness rather than analysed as behaviour appropriate to the violation, however long ago. If violating experiences are also more strongly associated with certain populations based on some characteristic or other, then collective responses to institutional authority including psychiatry are similarly comprehensible. The social determinants that we associate with health outcomes are also strongly associated with early life experiences and skills – the development of academic and social skills and confidence. These are tools that provide opportunities in the attainment of social mobility, key among them, the ability to 'fit in' with middle-class norms, values, and expectations. An exchange that facilitates some degree of acceptability and trust. Challenging family and neighbourhood backgrounds, regardless of adverse or abusive behaviour, tend to produce relatively defensive behaviours, a toughening up for what is perceived and experienced as a tough world. Such environments are more likely to generate relatively low self-confidence and mistrust compared to middle-class children, cognitive and emotional traits that are hard to dissolve as adults.

Compassion, empathy, and trust

Poor childhood attachment not only creates vulnerability for emotional mental health problems contingent on their accompaniment with various childhood adversities but also that it impacts on social relationships and connectedness with others. Mental illness, arguably much more than most physical illnesses, disrupts and damages social relationships, partially related to communication problems. For example, symptoms of schizophrenia are associated with abnormalities in thought, language, and speech; depression is sometimes accompanied by a 'shutting down'. Most people with a chronic or life-limiting illness experience a biographical disruption to their assumed understanding of their abilities and trajectories, obliging the individual to rethink their life and concept of self in fundamental ways, sometimes in terms of mortality. Drawing on Giddens' concept of a critical situation (Giddens, 1979) what emerges is a new consciousness of the body and existential fragility. Depending on the type and severity of the disability or illness, there may be difficulties negotiating relationships due to 'burden of care'. However, where there is no gross alteration of the individual's personality, relationships may be altered but maintain a general integrity. This situation can be every different for people living with schizophrenia, major depressive illnesses, or a neurological condition who have vastly more difficulty in grasping the biographical disruption but also have to deal with a biographical narrative that has no coherence where memories and their meanings are uncertain and fluid (Allé et al., 2015). As in Simmel's concept of the stranger, the person with the mental or neurological condition is simultaneously insider and outsider, known but unknowable. One of the most significant upsets reported by family members is that their loved one has somehow lost the essence of themselves – what gave them a unique identity. This sense of strangeness tends not be observed among families of people who develop a physical illness. The estrangement created by mental illness may also be supplemented by a decrease in caregiver compassion, a strain caused by the perceived loss of self.

The impoverishment of verbal and social skills means that the individual is less able to engage and cooperate effectively with others to mutual satisfaction. Their ability to respond appropriately and build friendships becomes imprisoning. Bowlby argues that humans have an inherent propensity for concern and caregiving for others, trust-building skills of empathy and compassion, even for those whom we are not intimately or socially connected. This caregiving blueprint, like secure attachment, is generated in childhood through an internalised working model. Interpersonal demonstration of empathy and compassion is commonly considered as altruistic; understood from an evolutionary perspective, such behaviour towards extended others who share the same genes may be seen as promoting survival of the group, leaving altruism less obvious or important.

Within attachment theory, the caregiving system opens a portal to the study of compassion and altruism; moreover, understanding this system provides a foundation for devising ways to increase people's compassion and effective altruism (Shaver et al., 2016, p. 879). As Shaver and colleagues suggest, the most salient aspect of the caregiving system is the external focus on the needs of others rather than an inward self-concern. Put simply, the twin operation of the attachment and caregiving system means that because the secure individual has received and internalised the sensitive attention of at least on parent, this ability is more accessible as an internalised working model and likely to be reproduced in the care of others. A secure individual's positive model of self provides a platform in the management of another's distress, while simultaneously coping successfully with their own emotions. A less secure individual may have empathic feelings regarding the distress of another person but unable to respond because of anxiety and thus, they are more likely to retreat to self-protection. According to Ainsworth and colleagues, anxiety and avoidance underpin various attachment patterns (Ainsworth et al., 2015). They may wish to respond, and will feel conflicted in not doing so, but are restrained by mistrust in the other and themselves.

Optimism

Optimism, generally conceptualised as a way of seeing the world, more generally, as benign, or the outcome of a specific situation or event, as turning out well. In this sense, it may be regarded as closely related but not the same as trust. Thus, it is more of a characteristic of the optimistic individual rather than how one regards the person to be trusted or mistrusted. Optimism has been theorised as influencing how individuals approach life and life events, including illness, and is believed to confer various protections such as having more salutogenic and positive attitudes, experiencing less stress and the ability to cope with difficulties (Conversano et al., 2010). However, it is also possible that optimists have a tendency towards misrecognition of potential harms, considered by some as a 'bias of self' (Weinstein, 1984) whereby the optimistic person underestimate the likelihood of a negative event for themselves but relatively elevates the risk for others. This kind of optimistic bias may not be a trait or inherent disposition, but rather due to limited information and poor self-assessment of personal cognitive skills. Alternatively, the optimistic bias may arise from the individual's need to protect self-esteem.

Other studies have shown pessimism to be correlated more highly with suicidal ideation than levels of depression and remained so, controlling for depression (Hirsch & Conner, 2006). Moreover, other researchers have suggested that the development of interventions to enhance optimism may help reduce suicidality in certain patients (Chochinov et al., 1998). Alternatively, it has been argued that people who have a pessimistic explanatory style – that is, consistent with the leamed helplessness experienced by people and animals developed during exposure to non-contingent events that outcomes will happen anyway, regardless of one own behaviour. Relatively fatalistic, pessimists may be at higher risk for depressive and anxiety disorders. It is also likely that such individuals experience challenges in navigating life, with severely restricted opportunities in various domains of life. Rather depressingly, Peterson and Seligman concluded that 'passivity, pessimism, and low morale foreshadow disease and death' (1987). Unfortunately, evidence from studies of optimism and mortality tends to support this assessment (Giltay et al., 2006; Yue et al., 2022). Optimists tend to see an adverse event as inconstant or, if unavoidable, will be able to manage them better, thus better armed with resilience and locus of control. If, as suggested by various commentators that pessimism and misguided optimism are learned cognitions and behaviours rather than inherent traits, then such dispositions can be 're-programmed', altered towards a more realistic and effective approach to managing life's challenges.

Loneliness, not be confused with being alone, is commonly defined as a subjective experience, a feeling that the quality of one's relationships is deficient, a perceived discrepancy between one's desired and actual relationships with others. Experimental evidence, in which feelings of loneliness were induced hypnotically induced, noted an increase in depressive symptoms, perceived stress, anxiety, and anger. What the researchers also found was that loneliness impacted negatively on the participant's self-evaluation and weakened their sense of optimism (Cacioppo et al., 2006).

Loneliness

One dimension of ontological insecurity that has strikingly caught the attention of social commentators, policy makers, and public health practitioners, regularly referred to as an epidemic and a public health issue, is loneliness. Bear in mind that this a 'problem' within highly developed, Western economies rather than rural and underdeveloped traditional societies. If loneliness is a problem in the latter, we don't know about it, probably because of competition with other concerns such as war and ecological devastation. Loneliness is also linked to various life-limiting physical health problems such as coronary heart disease, diabetes, and hypertension. It is often quoted, even by the United States Surgeon General that in mortality terms, loneliness is the equivalent of smoking 15 cigarettes a day (Office of the Surgeon, 2023). It has been implicated in the development of cognitive decline and dementia (Lazzari & Rabottini, 2022) and while not a diagnosable mental illness, it is also strongly associated with depression, self-harm, and suicide.

Emphasising the social dimension of human life, two of the foremost experts in the epidemiology of loneliness, Louise Hawkley and John Cacioppo, have posited an evolutionary significance for loneliness and the need for 'safe, secure social surround to survive and thrive' (Cacioppo et al., 2006; Hawkley & Cacioppo, 2010). Thus, feelings of loneliness are analogous to hunger, thirst, or physical pain caused by a wound, they alert human beings to a potential danger – a warning signal for vulnerability that should be attended to. The problem for many people who experience loneliness is that they fail to respond to the signals of discomfort. This sets off implicit hypervigilance for (additional) social threat in the environment. In Hawksley and Cacioppo's model, the perception of social isolation tends to trigger an 'unconscious surveillance' for threats in the environment. Lonely people who view the social world as threatening develop an anticipation of negative or hostile social experiences underpinned by negative memories or appraisals of events. In a vicious circle, the individual's anticipation and accompanying responses only serve to stimulate negative responses from others, thus confirming the lonely persons' expectations of a bad outcome. In this way, a self-fulfilling prophecy is established whereby potential social partners are avoided while simultaneously attributing the cause of the social distance to others. Pessimists and lonely people share a considerable level of passivity. The belief that nothing can be done about loneliness is related to the individual's external locus of control. While still, essentially, a defence mechanism, it is nevertheless a maladaptive way of coping with the world. Thus, the social destructiveness of loneliness is also found in the lonely individual's inability to self-regulate has considerable negative impacts on lifestyles and health behaviours. Socially isolated and lonely people have less healthy diets than non-lonely people and more likely to smoke and drink alcohol at higher levels. They also engage in much less physical activity than non-lonely people and are, therefore, less likely to receive the physical and mental health benefits that physical exercise confers.

There a wide range of situational factors associated with loneliness – poor mental health, physical disability, living alone, or being a migrant. While loneliness is commonly reported in the context of old age and the factors associated with getting old, retirement, bereavement, and so on, evidence suggests that younger people are just as likely as older people to experience loneliness, in some studies more so. Recent international evidence found that loneliness charted a non-linear trajectory with elevated levels in people aged 70 years or more and adults aged under 30 years (Hawkley et al., 2022; Luhmann & Hawkley, 2016; Victor & Yang, 2012).[1] Victor and Yang's (2012) study of European countries also noted higher levels of loneliness among Greek and post-Soviet Union bloc countries relative to Western European countries which may be explained by high migration rates of young people in search of work elsewhere, leaving older generations behind. It is impossible to state if greater levels of loneliness in the former Soviet Union countries are related to a breakdown in social cohesion and low levels of trust, but it is true that the dissolution of the old political system, the rapid assimilation of capitalism, and the complete absence of anything resembling a civic society would have done little to enhance interpersonal and generalised trust. In any case, it is difficult to disentangle the external macro-level socio-political contexts and their influence on micro-level and interpersonal circumstances.

Belonging and trust

While migration is well acknowledged as a risk factor for mental health problems, not everyone who migrates is at risk. Indeed, some migrant communities appear to fare much better than others for mental health outcomes. What puts migrants at risk of depression and other disorders are the events and circumstances prior to leaving their homeland, the challenges in the migration journey, and the reception and settlement experiences following arrival in the new country. The heterogeneity and complex interplay of protective and risk factors within and between each national migrant group, and in each migration context (country to country), ensures that there are no simple linear connections between the migration event and the potential for mental health problems. For educated, multi-lingual, and affluent migrants, transfer from one cosmopolitan elite milieu to another, the migration pathway and settlement, is likely to be smooth and will pose few challenges, unlike, their under resourced counterparts whose every step is risk-laden, difficult, and stressful. The opportunities, choices, and outcomes for each are unevenly distributed. While each migrant trusts that life will be better in the new country, or at least, a stepping stone to improvement, the level and significance of that trust differ hugely, and this is largely related to the circumstances, motivation, and expectations of the migrant and migrant group. Here, the contrast between economic 'migrant' and 'refugee' is somewhat ambiguous, as many so-called economic migrants are exposed to dangers and oppression that don't fit with conventional definitions of refugee criteria which can often rest on whether the migration act was voluntary or involuntary and the intentions of the migrant. The 'economic migrants' who travel long distances through South America to seek refuge in the United States are often fleeing from violence and hunger are a case in point. Poverty, sexual violence, and other adverse 'domestic' events rather than national events push many individuals towards exile but are not accepted as criteria for refugee status. Evidence of poor physical and mental health among Irish migrants living in the United Kingdom interested me. They appeared to be the only migrant group whose health outcomes remained lower relative to the British-born into the second and third generation (Harding & Balarajan, 1996). The Irish were predominantly white, spoke English, and travel between the two countries was relatively straightforward and inexpensive, involving no risky travel or visa entry. Moreover, large Irish communities had been settled in Britain for over a century, with recognisably high levels of social capital. Although various explanations for the poor mental health of Irish migrants included material deprivation, racism, cultural and lifestyle factors such as alcohol abuse, epidemiological research was limited (Commander et al., 1999).

Counterintuitively, we suggested that the geographical proximity to Britain and the associated increased likelihood of an unplanned migration posed mental health risks among Irish migrants in England. In a case-control study, we found that the hypothesis of an effect for unplanned migration on depression held true, but only for men, and noted protective factors among women that we had not considered, including gendered aspects of social support which mitigated against depression (Ryan et al., 2006).

The concept of the 'myth of return', previously examined in relation to older Pakistanis in the North of England, relates to the expectations of migrants to return to their country of origin, expectations which were generally unfulfilled, and which severely restricted participation in British institutions. Believing that settlement was temporary, they intended to save, invest, and eventually return 'home'. However, most remained in Britain due to economic factors and to remain with their children. Stuck between cultures and place, the first-generation migrants felt stranded in later life and experienced depression. Studies of Irish migrants reveal strong connections between adverse events in childhood, trust, loneliness, and mental health over the life course (Leavey, 2001). Thus, combined in the narratives of poverty pre-migration, many of the Irish migrants revealed dire adverse events including abuse, the death of parents in childhood, abandonment, and alienation that appears to have endured throughout their lives. Thus, unless diverted by distinct psychological resilience and socially protective factors, these childhood adversities influence various mutually reinforcing attitudes and behaviours that heighten risks for loneliness. Repressive attitudes to intimacy, an inability to connect meaningfully with others, resulted in maladaptive coping in the form of heavy alcohol use.

Migration for most is based on trust that 'things will be better' but a trust that is also supported by the material and symbolic evidence of migration success that is projected by previous migrant cohorts, but which, is often illusory. The affluence of the returning sojourner migrant although ephemeral was nevertheless convincing to people at home eager for change. It was not a generalised trust of the host country, a long historical familiarity in a relationship of conflict would suggest otherwise, but rather a trust based on a type of continuity with, and bounded by, one's community that exists elsewhere. That so many of these Irish migrants left without planning resonates with a kind of 'blind faith' trust. Thus, for males at least, the diaspora community provided a social capital that had its foundations within the institutions of the Catholic Church, public houses, and the construction industry. However, while the kind of social capital that emerges within the post-war Irish community migrants was aligned to the challenges of everyday life that they faced, it also had the potential to further undermine health and wellbeing. The men described an unsettled peripatetic life, dictated by the demands of work, squalid housing, and social isolation, devoid of long-term and intimate relations. They described themselves as extremely shy and had difficulty in forming relationships. The Irish public houses provided a hub for information about jobs and accommodation but as a panacea to loneliness was harmful. We may consider cultural behaviours and attitudes such as acceptance of heavy drinking, and a strict, religiously inspired sexual suppression, as evidence of psychosocial explanations for poor health, but this is insufficient. What also emerges from these narratives of the migrant experience is the commonly articulated complex and difficult relationship that depressed and lonely individuals have with home and family (as represented by Ireland) which in many behavioural aspects resemble attachment problems. If voluntary action is an inherent aspect of trust requiring the individual to have agency (the capacity to think, plan, and act), then what is the status of trust in the migration event? To some extent, this depends on our interpretation of agency, its constraints, and the available choices. As with most migrants, the sense of threat to one's life can be immediate, as in the belief that violence and death may be imminent or it may be the gradual feeling of a 'slow' death, a future emptied of prospects, a mistrust of the present, or an expectation of a better life. The issue of coercion may seem academic in the context.

Trust and loneliness in the digital age

Loneliness as an expression of disconnectedness in the digital era of hyper-communication and connectedness appears counterintuitive. The use of digital platforms and social media means that people can be in contact with many people over time and space. Except of course, whereby lonely people, regardless of proximity and form of meeting and presence (online or in-person), still anticipate a negative response from others and are unable to alter their state of loneliness through any type of connection.

The largest survey of loneliness undertaken by the BBC in the United Kingdom indicated that young people aged 16 to 24 years' experience loneliness more often and more intensely than other age groups. Like many such surveys, the data were collected from a self-selecting rather than random, sample, leaving questions about validity and representativeness. The size of the sample, nevertheless, helps to lessen some of the methodological concerns and the findings are intriguing. For example, there were no differences between in the amount of time given by lonely people and non-lonely people to use social media but the usage itself is quite different. Lonely people have more Facebook friends, but these remain distant and tend not to be 'real-life friends'. Again, lonely people reported lower levels of trust. In combination, these data suggest while the internet is a potential tool for increasing sociability and social contact, lonely people tend not to use it in this way.

While some people use the internet to reach out to others, maintain or expand their networks, others may find its various social platforms as a more convenient way of retreating from threatening social engagement while ameliorating the shame and low self-esteem that accompanies many lonely people. In a sense, this is a bad bargain. Thus, internet use may afford a greater degree of propping up low self-esteem relative to lonely people who don't use it, but it remains a weak strategy. For people who are potentially but not quite lonely, the use of social technologies can facilitate a drift into the displacement of 'real friendships' and communications. The relationship between loneliness and the use of social media platforms may be contingent on motivation although the concept of motivation as a means of managing anxiety implies something quite deliberate and conscious, when the opposite is more likely. A longitudinal study showed that Facebook use to develop friendships reduced peer-related loneliness over time, while using Facebook as a means of social skills compensation and reducing feelings of loneliness, increased peer-related loneliness over time (Teppers et al., 2014).[2]

While making the connection between loneliness and mistrust in the development of mental health problems, we should note the additional damage created by social isolation and poor social support, loneliness's companion. Loneliness and socially isolation have much in common and as concepts, may be overlapping; the main difference is that people may be socially isolated but do not feel lonely. For many others, loneliness is a consequence of isolation which may be caused by place – residence in remote and rural areas or circumstances such as age, migration, disability, relationship breakdown, or bereavement. The lack of social support increases the vulnerability of individuals to poor physical and mental health through lower physical activity, poor diet, and the misuse of alcohol and cigarettes as a way of managing stress and depression. Without the presence and vigilance of significant others in close proximity or regular contact, psychic and physical deterioration are more likely to go unnoticed or deterred. The presence of a caregiver allows for the possibility of confrontation and change but also opportunity for help-seeking and health interventions. When a medical intervention has been triggered, informal caregivers can then provide affective and instrumental support such as encouraging adherence to treatment, arranging and attending medical consultations, and monitoring improvement or deterioration. This level of support can make all the difference between early intervention and recovery or a poor pathway into care, or a prolonged, problematic relationship with psychiatric services, often with regular involuntary admissions to hospital.

There is however, a counterargument to the popular concern that there is too much loneliness in society, and that is, we have lost the capacity to be alone, that we suffer from a chronic overload of social contact and connectedness (Svensden, 2017). Both positions can be true. While many people feel liberated by technology, its affordance of shifting tasks in time and space, there is also the oppressive anxiety that technology provides an omnipresent intrusion of work and other sectors into one's privacy and private time, a boundaryless, continuous external vigilance prompting a hypervigilance that we may have missed something. It is also true that because we live longer, we are more likely to spend more of our time living with loss and things that make us lonely, disability, and cultural alienation, for example.

Alienation and suicide

Globally, over 700,000 people a year die by suicide, although this is probably an underestimate as in many parts of the world, it remains underreported for religious and cultural reasons (WHO, 2021). Suicide is a complex interplay between individual and social factors over the life course and the main risk factors are often common, making an accurate detection of suicidality by clinicians hard to detect, even though most people who die will have seen a family doctor in the 12 months prior to death (Leavey et al., 2016). Many suicides occur, according to relatives and friends, as completely 'out of the blue', a shockingly spontaneous and unpredictable action. Nevertheless, we have a crude understanding of the profile of suicides in that the evidence indicates most are male[3] and many have a history of mental health problems. In many cases, alcohol use was detected. Socio-economic difficulties related to unemployment, financial debt, and homelessness appear to contribute to an increased risk of suicide. These factors hint at pre-existing problems but challenges that are common to many people but cannot indicate why this person is suicidal and not another.

Suicide, as Camus noted in Sisyphus, 'is the only serious philosophical question', directing us to the meaning and purpose of existence. Simultaneously, an intensely private act but with social meaning and impact, it is almost impossible to ascertain what the individual was thinking in the hours, minutes, and seconds prior to the action that led to death. For some, premeditating factors can be assessed because they left behind a written explanation or provided one after surviving a suicide attempt. Hopelessness as an emotional state is defined by a lack, or absence, of optimism. At its core, suicidality is a loss of trust in self, others, and fortune that there is a non-suicidal solution to the perceived or actual source of the person's suffering.

Durkheim's analysis of national and regional variation and consistency in suicide rates led him to hypothesise the important role of social integration and anomie. National or group solidarity provided a protective bulwark against suicide 'egoistic' characterised by an individual's social disconnection, or 'anomic', defined crudely here as a failure or breakdown of social norms. The latter, of course, marked by massive change wrought by industrialisation and urbanisation provides the context for Durkheim's theory on suicide. Whether anomic or egoistic, Durkheim viewed suicide as the consequence of social isolation, an alienation from society and social norms. I use the term 'alienation' carefully here, not intending any confusion with Marx's use of the concept which refers to a separation of workers from the objects they create and over which they have no intellectual and emotional connection, a situation brought about by capitalist processes. The customary hesitancy in using the term relates to its quite fluid meaning but is imbued with a quality which in the context of social isolation and suicide feels correct. Thus, alienation or estrangement (*entfremdung*), commonly described as a key feature of modernity, has been employed to suggest an emotional disconnection from places or people that are, or should be, significant to the individual. While alienation may include family, peers, or work, the disconnection with one's sense of self is often cause or effect. This also extends to, resonates with, and possibly reinforced by pervasive feelings of meaningless in life that there is purposeless in self or the direction of humanity, politics, or indeed, the planet. Alienation may also refer to feelings of powerlessness and lack of autonomy that one's situation and life chances are externally controlled or the individual's personal impotence to effect change at an interpersonal or wider political level. In this sense, alienation may additionally reflect a high degree of cultural disconnection with social values and norms that these make little sense to the individual or are in opposition to new and evolved social ideas. The thematic areas covered by alienation or estrangement may be combined and mutually reinforcing. Individuals may struggle temporarily with feelings of alienation in specific age or place contexts; for example, the early experiences of a migrant from a rural background now living in a city or the feelings that often accompany the transition from adolescence to adulthood, precarious jobs, or negotiating an alien ideology.

When alienation is profound and enduring, the individual's social disconnection is usually generalised and total in that the compartmentalisation of disengagement with specific life domains seems unlikely. It is also accompanied by strong emotions such as unhappiness or anger. In either case, the individual experiences social isolation and a sense of meaninglessness. In its widest sense, this isolation refers to an anomic detachment from society and societal norms; in its more specific sense, it refers to an isolation from the individual's primary groups, that is, family, community, and work groups who may be, potentially at least, a bridge to the protective sanity offered by society. However, the hopelessness which in itself constitutes a loss of social trust is in many cases the by-product of social rejection experienced by the suicidal individual, whether this is some form of violent behaviour or the exclusion and despair created by structural violence.

Notes

1   Hawkley et al. (2016) note that minority ethnic groups were underrepresented across the adult age range, partly explained by selective mortality underprivileged African American adults. That they are 'missing' from the older age groups may be a survivor effect in that minority groups also record as lonelier, with loneliness increasing the risk for mortality.
2   The evidence that for a relationship between time spent on internet use and mental health problems is often weak or contradictory. Many such studies are cross-sectional and have considerable methodological weaknesses, not least in terms of measurement and limitations related to socio-economic and socio-demographic confounding factors. While time spent on the internet may be relatively obtainable, motivations in usage is more problematic, as is the content and sites used.
3   Suicide rates are estimated to be 9.4 per 100,000 for all persons (95% CI 8.5–10.3); males (13.3 per 100,000 [11.3–14.7]) and females (5.7 per 100,000 [5.1–6.4]).

References

Ainsworth, M. D. S., Blehar, M. C., Waters, E., & Wall, S. N. (2015). *Patterns of attachment: A psychological study of the strange situation.* Psychology Press.

Allé, M. C., Potheegadoo, J., Köber, C., Schneider, P., Coutelle, R., Habermas, T., Danion, J. M., & Berna, F. (2015). Impaired coherence of life narratives of patients with schizophrenia. *Scientific Reports, 5,* 12934. https://doi.org/10.1038/srep12934

Berger, P., & Luckman, T. (1966). *The social construction of reality.* Doubleday.

Bretherton, I. (1985). Attachment theory: Retrospect and prospect. *Monographs of the Society for Research in Child Development, 50*(1/2), 3–35. https://doi.org/10.2307/3333824

Cacioppo, J. T., Hawkley, L. C., Ernst, J. M., Burleson, M., Berntson, G. G., Nouriani, B., & Spiegel, D. (2006). Loneliness within a nomological net: An evolutionary perspective. *Journal of Research in Personality, 40*(6), 1054–1085.

Cassidy, J. (2016). The nature of the child's ties. In J. Cassidy & P. R. Shaver (Eds.), *Handbook of attachment: Theory, research, and clinical applications* (3rd ed.). Guilford Press.

CDC. (2008). *Child maltreatment surveillance: Uniform definitions for public health and recommended data elements.* Centers for Disease Control and Prevention, National Center for Injury Prevention and Control.

Chochinov, H. M., Wilson, K. G., Enns, M., & Lander, S. (1998). Depression, hopelessness, and suicidal ideation in the terminally ill. *Psychosomatics, 39*(4), 366–370. https://doi.org/10.1016/s0033-3182(98)71325-8

Commander, M., Odell, S., Sashidharan, S., & Surtees, P. (1999). Psychiatric morbidity in people born in Ireland. *Social Psychiatry and Psychiatric Epidemiology, 34,* 565–569.

Conversano, C., Rotondo, A., Lensi, E., Della Vista, O., Arpone, F., & Reda, M. A. (2010). Optimism and its impact on mental and physical well-being. *Clinical Practice and Epidemiology in Mental Health, 6,* 25–29. https://doi.org/10.2174/1745017901006010025

Danese, A., & McEwen, B. S. (2012). Adverse childhood experiences, allostasis, allostatic load, and age-related disease. *Physiology & Behavior, 106*(1), 29–39. https://doi.org/10.1016/j.physbeh.2011.08.019

Frewen, P. A., & Lanius, R. A. (2006). Toward a psychobiology of posttraumatic self-dysregulation: Reexperiencing, hyperarousal, dissociation, and emotional numbing. *Annals of the New York Academy of Sciences, 1071*, 110–124. https://doi.org/10.1196/annals.1364.010

Giddens, A. (1979). Central problems in social theory: Action, structure and contradictions in social analysis. University of California Press.

Giltay, E. J., Kamphuis, M. H., Kalmijn, S., Zitman, F. G., & Kromhout, D. (2006). Dispositional optimism and the risk of cardiovascular death: The Zutphen elderly study. *Archives of Internal Medicine, 166*(4), 431–436. https://doi.org/10.1001/archinte.166.4.431

Harding, S., & Balarajan, R. (1996). Patterns of mortality in second generation Irish living in England and Wales: Longitudinal study. *British Medical Journal, 312*(7043), 1389–1392.

Hawkley, L. C., Buecker, S., Kaiser, T., & Luhmann, M. (2022). Loneliness from young adulthood to old age: Explaining age differences in loneliness. *International Journal of Behavioral Development, 46*(1), 39–49. https://doi.org/10.1177/0165025420971048

Hawkley, L. C., & Cacioppo, J. T. (2010). Loneliness matters: A theoretical and empirical review of consequences and mechanisms. *Annals of Behavioral Medicine, 40*(2), 218–227. https://doi.org/10.1007/s12160-010-9210-8

Hirsch, J. K., & Conner, K. R. (2006). Dispositional and explanatory style optimism as potential moderators of the relationship between hopelessness and suicidal ideation. *Suicide and Life-Threatening Behavior, 36*(6), 661–669. https://doi.org/10.1521/suli.2006.36.6.661

Hughes, K., Bellis, M. A., Hardcastle, K. A., Sethi, D., Butchart, A., Mikton, C., Jones, L., & Dunne, M. P. (2017). The effect of multiple adverse childhood experiences on health: A systematic review and meta-analysis. *Lancet Public Health, 2*(8), e356–e366. https://doi.org/10.1016/s2468-2667(17)30118-4

Lazzari, C., & Rabottini, M. (2022). COVID-19, loneliness, social isolation and risk of dementia in older people: A systematic review and meta-analysis of the relevant literature. *International Journal of Psychiatry in Clinical Practice, 26*(2), 196–207. https://doi.org/10.1080/13651501.2021.1959616

Leavey, G. (2001). Too close for comfort: Mental illness and the Irish in Britain. In D. Bhugra & R. Littlewood (Eds.), *Colonialism and psychiatry*. Oxford University Press.

Leavey, G., Rosato, M., Galway, K., Hughes, L., Mallon, S., & Rondon, J. (2016). Patterns and predictors of help seeking contacts with health services and general practice detection of suicidality. *BMC Psychiatry, 16*(1), 120.

Luhmann, M., & Hawkley, L. C. (2016). Age differences in loneliness from late adolescence to oldest old age. *Developmental Psychology, 52*(6), 943.

Moog, N. K., Cummings, P. D., Jackson, K. L., Aschner, J. L., Barrett, E. S., Bastain, T. M., Blackwell, C. K., Bosquet Enlow, M., Breton, C. V., Bush, N. R., Deoni, S. C. L., Duarte, C. S., Ferrara, A., Grant, T. L., Hipwell, A. E., Jones, K., Leve, L. D., Lovinsky-Desir, S., Miller, R. K., ..., Buss, C. (2023). Intergenerational transmission of the effects of maternal exposure to childhood maltreatment in the USA: A retrospective cohort study. *Lancet Public Health, 8*(3), e226–e237. https://doi.org/10.1016/s2468-2667(23)00025-7

Office of the Surgeon, G. (2023). *Publications and reports of the surgeon general. In our epidemic of loneliness and isolation: The U.S. Surgeon General's advisory on the healing effects of social connection and community*. US Department of Health and Human Services.

Peterson, C., & Seligman, M. E. (1987). Explanatory style and illness. *Journal of Personality, 55*(2), 237–265. https://doi.org/10.1111/j.1467-6494.1987.tb00436.x

Rothbaum, F., Weisz, J., Pott, M., Miyake, K., & Morelli, G. (2000). Attachment and culture. Security in the United States and Japan. *American Psychologist, 55*(10), 1093–1104. https://doi.org/10.1037//0003-066x.55.10.1093

Ryan, L., Leavey, G., Golden, A., Blizard, R., & King, M. (2006). Depression in Irish migrants living in London: Case-control study. *The British Journal of Psychiatry, 188*(6), 560–566.

Shaver, P. R., Mikulinter, M., Gross, J. T., Stern, J., & Cassidy, J. (2016). A lifespan perspective on attachment; empathy, altruism and prosocial behaviour. In J. Cassidy & P. R. Shaver (Eds.), *Handbook of attachment; theory, research and clinical applications*. The Guilford Press.

Su, S., Jimenez, M. P., Roberts, C. T., & Loucks, E. B. (2015). The role of adverse childhood experiences in cardiovascular disease risk: A review with emphasis on plausible mechanisms. *Current Cardiology Reports, 17*(10), 88. https://doi.org/10.1007/s11886-015-0645-1

Svensden, L. (2017). *A philosophy of loneliness*. Reaktion Books.

Teicher, M. H., Andersen, S. L., Polcari, A., Anderson, C. M., & Navalta, C. P. (2002). Developmental neurobiology of childhood stress and trauma. *Psychiatric Clinics of North America, 25*(2), 397–426, vii-viii. https://doi.org/10.1016/s0193-953x(01)00003-x

Teicher, M. H., Andersen, S. L., Polcari, A., Anderson, C. M., Navalta, C. P., & Kim, D. M. (2003). The neurobiological consequences of early stress and childhood maltreatment. *Neuroscience & Biobehavioral Reviews, 27*(1–2), 33–44. https://doi.org/10.1016/s0149-7634(03)00007-1

Teppers, E., Luyckx, K., Klimstra, T. A., & Goossens, L. (2014). Loneliness and Facebook motives in adolescence: A longitudinal inquiry into directionality of effect. *Journal of Adolescence, 37*(5), 691–699. https://doi.org/10.1016/j.adolescence.2013.11.003

Victor, C. R., & Yang, K. (2012). The prevalence of loneliness among adults: A case study of the United Kingdom. *The Journal of Psychology, 146*(1–2), 85–104.

Weinstein, N. D. (1984). Why it won't happen to me: Perceptions of risk factors and susceptibility. *Health Psychology, 3*(5), 431.

WHO. (2021). *Suicide worldwide in 2019: Global health estimates*. World Health Organization Geneva.

Yue, Z., Liang, H., Qin, X., Ge, Y., Xiang, N., & Liu, E. (2022). Optimism and survival: Health behaviors as a mediator – a ten-year follow-up study of Chinese elderly people. *BMC Public Health, 22*(1), 670. https://doi.org/10.1186/s12889-022-13090-3

Chapter 5

Adolescence, Vulnerability, and Trust

Something must be at stake to place trust in another person, an acceptance of risk for the encounter to be meaningful. In this chapter, I argue that the significant object at risk for an adolescent is a potential loss of sense of agency, esteem and autonomy, to be regarded as a competent person, capable of managing their own affairs. However, the period of adolescence, transitioning to adulthood tends to be experienced as a liminal space, where the person is regarded in most cultures as neither fully child nor fully adult, and as the evidence suggests, is a difficult period. To seek help from a parent or other adult is an admission of vulnerability which many young people will be loath to do, despite the high help seeking preference ratings that parents are generally accorded in youth surveys. To be regarded as vulnerable invites a new and unwanted status as having needs and/or needing protection, even when this is reasonable and well intentioned, at a point in life when independence and agency have such significance, at least among young people.

Adolescence

Situated somewhere between childhood and adulthood, adolescence is considered a transitional stage in which physiological, hormonal, and psychological changes combine to provoke considerable turbulence, insecurity, and anxiety. For some time, adolescence or youth was considered as little more than a 20th-century Western social construct, characterised by surly teenage behaviour. However, new scientific knowledge on brain maturation and physical development indicates that following infancy, adolescence is a second period of rapid development and learning. Changes in the brain are rapidly accompanied by a pubertal growth spurt, metabolic changes, and alteration to sleep and circadian rhythms.

Concurrently, sexual maturation through hormonal and genital development also produces change in body hair, skin, and muscle growth. It is a stage where trust in self and the world is thoroughly tested. The hormonal and physiological changes propel the individual towards a more fully expressed sexual maturity but are generally lacking the emotional literacy that can help shape healthy and informed decision-making. Paradoxically, this comes at a time when emotional literacy is crucial to wellbeing, and in some cases, survival. Simply put, adolescents seek

DOI: 10.4324/9781003326687-5

greater social extra-familial connections, and are motivated towards risk-taking and sensation-seeking, and highly conscious of social status and peer evaluation. Sexual interest emerges alongside the challenges, for some, of grappling with sexual orientation and tastes. Many Western families will recognise adolescence as a period of withdrawal from family life, an inchoate, sometimes incoherent need for separation from parents. In non-Western and traditional societies, there are more formal rites of passage that conduct the young person into adulthood – anthropology describes these transitional experiences as liminal – from the Latin word *limen,* meaning threshold. This is an intense period of ambiguity and ontological insecurity – a state of being neither one thing or another, neither child nor adult, the individual requires a settled identity and place but commonly feels stranded and alone. Similarly, in Western societies, young people seek to establish an identity and in doing so, often place themselves at a distance from family and family values and interests. This period of alienation can be distressing for young people and their families. Commonly, it typifies an individuation process, a normal developmental outworking of physiological and psychological change. When the alienation suggests something more potentially serious and deteriorating, the seclusion arising from mistrust will have consequences for the search for meaning and help, ultimately.

Cognitive skills and risk-taking in adolescence

Adolescence produces considerable change in the executive function of the brain, with rapid enhancement of cognitive skills that assist control and coordination of one's thoughts and behaviours. Such changes are thought to have enduring influence into adulthood, crucially determining illness and responses to it. Of major relevance to trust and trust behaviours, up to adolescence, children's thinking tends to be concrete, rooted in present realties rather than an ability to consider alternative possibilities. As described by Bowlby and others, the child may be operating in a trustworthy (or untrustworthy) family environment in which the ability to engage with parents and others is relatively relaxed and stress-free (or not), an engagement that is taken for granted, an unpremeditated reflex. In this situation, vulnerability is not a consideration and there is no calculation of trust.

Trust as a recognisable concept comes to the fore as we transition to adolescence which brings more opportunities for choice and decision-making, coinciding as they do with an increased need for planning and strategising, reflecting on causes and weighing up the consequences of actions. In other words, they begin to build hypothetical and high-level probabilistic thinking – what is at stake? What are the consequences for me and others resulting from this or that action. While these cognitive skills which permit extended abstract reasoning provide more sophisticated reasoning about interpersonal relationships, beliefs, values, and morals, there is also the ability for self-reflection or mentalisation – 'theory of mind' which permits the individual to stand outside oneself – to think about one's thoughts, but also to think about what other people may be thinking. While these, undoubtedly, are important skills that assist social negotiation and autonomy, they also contain the potential for self-consciousness, social anxiety, and vulnerability. In many an adolescent's life, this is the constant struggle between self-development and annihilation. Risk-taking tends to be minimal in childhood but then accelerates between puberty and late adolescence to early adulthood, declining in adulthood (Reyna et al., 2011).

Although adolescent risk-taking elicits much social concern, or opprobrium, Reyna and Farley use a Life-span Wisdom Model of risk-taking, offering a more positive perspective that emphasises the useful, sometimes necessary, experience obtained through exploration in this phase of life. Thus, adolescent sensation-seeking is often driven by valuable environmental exploration, behaviour that must be distinguished from impulsive action, usually maladaptive, and many adolescents in Western societies engage in actions which imperil their health, education, careers, and sometimes their lives. Under ideal conditions (e.g., without temptations of high rewards and individual variances that diminish self-control) adolescents can make rational, goal-oriented decisions (2006). However, few humans operate in a strictly rational, calculative manner, quite often immediacy, pleasure-seeking, and emotion will trump deferred long-term benefits. Moreover, in sub-optimal conditions – being acquiescent in a large group, peer pressure to engage in risky behaviour, using inhibition-lowering substances, or experiencing depression – one's executive performance may be compromised, with poor outcomes. Young people with positive self-esteem and self-trust are less vulnerable to emotional and psychological distress, and external influences to engaging in high-risk behaviour. Although public health evidence tends to address and report these issues separately, we know that poor mental health, poor diet, substance misuse, and teenage pregnancy, among other problems, are usually not compartmentalised but rather are often mutually exacerbating components of similar origin and attempting to address discrete elements is rather pointless.

Adolescent mental health

It is a difficult time to be an adolescent and it seems to be getting worse. Even prior to the COVID 19 pandemic and the economic downturn, the evidence from mental health and hospital surveys consistently suggested that young people were far from happy. Across most Western countries there has been a considerable increase in various emotional and psychological disorders, and particularly noticeable rises in anxiety and depression among girls and young women. Approximately 15% of young people aged 10 to 19 years, globally, experience a mental health disorder. In our study of in Northern Ireland almost a quarter of females recorded a mental health problem more than twice that for males. Further, in the previous 12 months prior to the study, one-fifth had thought seriously about harming themselves (females, 27.1%; males, 11.1%) and 15% had thought about taking their own lives (Leavey et al., 2020). In the United Kingdom, among children and adolescents aged 7 to 16 years, rates rose by more than 4% in 3 years to 16.7% in 2020. In the same period, among those aged 17 to 19 years, rates of a probable mental disorder rose by more than 7% to 17.7% and rising again by 2022. In the United States, rates of depression and anxiety have also risen sharply in the past decade with suicidal behaviours among high school students increasing by more than 40% between 2010 and 2019 and suicide rates for young people aged 12 to 17 years increasing from 3.7 per 100,000 population to 6.3 per 100,000 population. Suicide is the second leading cause of death for young people aged 10 to 14 years; and the third leading cause of death of those aged 15 to 24 years.

It is impossible to pin down some single factor that explains these increases in adolescent mental health problems, indeed some people dispute an actual increase but instead show how good our healthcare systems have become in identifying problems and/or perhaps attributed to a gradual decrease in the stigma associated with mental illness, a greater societal openness to individual disclosure, and an improved capacity of individuals and families to recognise problems and seek help. All positive trends. Others argue that while certain diagnostic categories such as autism and Attention Deficit Hyperactivity Disorders (ADHD) are now increasingly recognised and treated by services (Thomas et al., 2015), the prevalence of major depression has remained fairly constant (Richter et al., 2019). Alternatively, Western societies have undergone through economic and political turmoil, to which problems can be added the omnipresent existential threat that is climate change. Young people in most Western democracies have expressed a sense of betrayal by a system organised by the older generations, that is perceived to be not acting in their interests and leaving a legacy of alienation and mistrust. In this context, why wouldn't we expect exponential increases in stress and anxiety in our children? Perhaps, as some experts have suggested, we might be too obsessed about an increased prevalence in psychological problems among younger people, rather than considering that most of them appear to be leading reasonably happy and fulfilling lives, or at least, not in need of psychiatric help, despite considerable adversities. Nevertheless, the upward trends in poor mental health are often accompanied by objectively measured behaviours such as self-harm, suicide attempts, and suicides, less easily dismissed as changed cultural perspectives on the nature of distress. With such similar trends across measures and settings, the weight of evidence indicates that adolescent mental health has deteriorated in recent decades.

The internet and adolescent mental health problems

Various studies of risk factors associated with adolescent psychological distress report exam stress and bullying. However, these factors are not new. A more plausible explanation is the growth of the internet, the ubiquitous use of smartphones and social media. There is now a considerable body of evidence that heavy social media use is linked, among other problems, to loneliness, anxiety, and suicidality (Lin et al., 2016; Riehm et al., 2019; Shensa et al., 2017). Although most such studies have been cross-sectional, and thus unable to determine cause or consequence, there is some evidence from more experimental studies pointing to a negative impact (Brailovskaia et al., 2022; Tromholt, 2016). Again, there are no singular and obvious explanatory mechanisms why this should be. It may be the psychological cost of lost or diminished social connections, time spent on social media is at the expense of being with friends and family which we know is beneficial to wellbeing.[1] Although we continue to explore the potential of the internet and social media as sources of an ever-expanding range of social, ethical, and psychological issues, the evidence remains ambiguous. Nevertheless, the impact on some children's mental health by cyber-bullying and the maleficent intentions of actors and internet sites promoting nihilist worldviews, self-harm, and suicide, is certain and worthy of further scrutiny. There have been several systematic reviews that highlight associations between social media and internet use and various adverse health risk behaviours including risky sexual activity, gambling, alcohol use, and smoking (Marino et al., 2018; Purba et al., 2023).[2] What is perhaps an obvious point in this discussion but one that is often forgotten, is that while social media allows wide connections and alternative normative perspectives on ideas and behaviour that may be illegal or simply disdained by older people, the internet provides easy and anonymous access to harmful goods and services. While the internet may be a portal to help-seeking, much help-seeking can be directed towards destructive ends and means. Thus, much less is known about why or how certain children connect to sites that have content on deliberate self-harm and suicide (Sedgwick et al., 2019). Young people may visit out of morbid but harmless curiosity or seek to understand their own difficult feelings and behaviours. Certainly, we know that high internet use is correlated with loneliness and depression among young people (Teppers et al., 2014).

The internet has many sites which offer self-help support, advice and guidance, some offer refuge for people who experience loneliness as 'outsiders' for this or that reason – a simple escape from isolation. The darker side of the internet, perhaps understandably, attracts most media and policy attention, possibly because it coincides with a growing concern about the seemingly unconstrained power of the major digital corporations and their harvesting of masses of data related to human interests and behaviours for commercial exploitation. While national governments across the globe fear and mistrust digital multinational corporations because of their ability to escape policy restraint and taxation, there is also justifiable unease about their ability to distance themselves from ethical and legal responsibilities as publishers of text and other materials. Such concerns have been highlighted by the suicide of children following contact with self-harm and suicide sites and forums (Marchant et al., 2018). What is picked up in this case is adolescent fragility in the establishment of the self, the upheaval and uncertainty in the transition to adulthood in which existential concerns begin to emerge. The emotional pain is often accompanied by a distancing from family and a retreat into bedrooms that now host the infinite space of the internet and access to sites which may hold the answer to teenage questions about identity and being. Powerful algorithms can take users immediately to a labyrinth of communities of like-minded teenagers and while most are helpful, many are devoted to often incoherent nihilistic philosophy, others lead to guidance and advice on self-harm and concealment. Other sites provide information on suicide sometimes accompanied by graphic material on methods. Meanwhile, chat rooms are busy with text from people directly encouraging others to suicide. While this phenomenon is of interest to research and policymakers, it is worth bearing in mind too that young people are reaching out to internet sites and communities to seek help from or meet their needs, however problematically or negatively slanted the fulfilment may be. Further, given the intergenerational cultural shifts in Western societies towards a more liberal form of parenting that have occurred over the past half-century, the rejection of parental support and help by their adolescent children may appear puzzling.

Sources of truth and knowledge

Whether there are truly increasing rates of mental health problems among young people or if these increases are due to increased symptom recognition is difficult to state definitively. First, it has been an easy observation that the rise in emotional and psychological illness among young people in advanced capitalist systems has emerged in the context of growing affluence – in general population terms, wealth does not purchase greater happiness or reduce anxiety. Despite the abundant freedoms that young people in western contexts have, relative to previous generations, they seem to be in less control of their lives and more fearful of the future. Given the imperilling of the planet through climate change, this is perhaps understandable, but the existential threats that are associated with adolescent distress may be more proximal. There are well-acknowledged perennial determinants of mental illness, particularly adverse childhood circumstances and events such as abuse, neglect, poverty, parental mental health and while these have some explanatory value for the increases witnessed in recent years, it may be difficult to argue that these are on the increase. Alternatively, the burgeoning power of the internet and social media has been linked by many commentators to a diverse range of harmful behaviours, psychological and social. Before touching on these putative harms, it should be stated that following every technological advance is a cacophony announcing all that is good and decent in society – radio and television have had their immediate and long-standing detractors that these media will turn the brains of our children to mush and civilisation to its knees. Previously, powerful religious forces railed against the printing press and the individual's access to learning. Thus, the apparent democratisation and ease of access to information creates anxiety among diverse conservative institutions and vested interests which see a dilution of their monopoly and power.

What worries many politicians and civic society is that the internet permeates all zones of human activity in ways that were unanticipated and exposes children to content that is relatively unregulated by government. For many people, the perceived benefits of the internet and the digital economy have universally blinded governments to the potential risks and harms, and the multinational organisations that dominate it have been allowed to pursue unbridled wealth creation heedless of the potential damage to society and particularly, the wellbeing of children and young people. This perspective holds that a barely vetted flood of toxic material threatens to engulf and psychologically damage. Additionally, while bullying behaviour is hardly a modern behaviour, it was generally restricted in the scale of intimacy and situation. The internet and social media permit a mass penetration of public humiliation and hurt, potentially without limits in time and place. There is nowhere that the bullied individual can hide. In a recent UK study (Newlove-Delgado et al., 2022) children aged 11 to 16 years with a probable mental disorder were more likely to have been bullied and less likely to feel safe in their neighbourhood or trust the people in that neighbourhood.

A different kind of conformity

Moreover, there are increasing concerns about the destabilising influence of the internet on human relationships. Social media platforms produce sophisticated, highly targeted advertising designed to arrest the attention of individuals, stimulating needs and anxieties with the aim of selling goods and services. Other social media provide images of what it is to be beautiful, exciting, popular, and successful, so ludicrously unobtainable that most people competing in this market for the perfect look, or the perfect partner are destined to 'fail' in the struggle to emulate the influencers. Previous generations in Western societies contended mostly with moral frameworks set by their parents, and with some adjustments, those of their grandparents. The immediate world of neighbourhood was a relatively unchanging one with limited exposure to outside influences, even after the major social liberalisation of the 1960s. By contrast, digital communication has saturated the worlds of younger individuals without regard to parental values and beliefs, permitting access into private spaces almost without limit. For many, this has become a surrender of guardianship in the service of amoral multinational corporations which claim a disinterest in anything other than harvesting as much data as it is possible to consume and analyse for the purpose of commercial marketing.

The consequences for child and adolescent mental health may be considerable. In addition to the rise in the prevalence of anxiety and depression, there is increasing evidence of eating disorders among young people, a range of problems characterised by a desire to lose weight and driven by anxieties about their weight, shape, size, and body image. Anorexia nervosa is currently prevalent in about 1 in every 200 adolescent girls, while 1% to 5% of their peers meet the criteria for bulimia nervosa. While once considered a culture-bound disorder and the domain of educated, middle-class Western females, eating disorders have moved beyond these perceived borders and are now found in minority ethnic groups and young men. Thus, the cultural ideal for women's body size and shape is now significantly lean and thinner while for men it is one of conditioned strength and muscularity. While the evidence of media influence on body image is often limited to qualitative and cross-sectional studies, it is difficult to refute the associations between media content, the target audience, and the outcome, intended or otherwise.

Once hidden among top-shelves and seedy shops, the pornography industry has exceptionally benefitted from the internet and easily accessed by young people, for whom it is argued, a considerable damage is done to emotional and psychological health. It does this in various ways. First, some evidence from a wide range of pornography users points to an addictive dimension, in which pornography watching is easily switched off by the individual but rather begins to dominate one's life, consuming increasing time, and a dose-response quality that demands material of increasing 'extremity'. Addictive pornography consumption may lead to or exacerbate existing adolescent isolation and loneliness. Interestingly, in addition to the obvious sexual gratification that pornography offers, users also suggest that pornography is used to cope with anxiety, stress, and depression (Bridges & Morokoff, 2011; Willoughby et al., 2016; Wright et al., 2017). Second, there is a negative impact on body and sexuality self-perceptions – tapping into adolescents' anxieties about their bodies and sexual performance. Additionally, sexual objectification is a key feature within the pornographic industry, in which women tend to be portrayed as passive objects for male sexual pleasure (Stewart & Szymanski, 2012). The idealised but typically misogynistic behaviour of the actors reinforces ideas of male dominance over women, and the often violent and abusive activities of male performers, has the effect of normalising such behaviours among actual adolescent relationships to the extent that female strangulation and other physical assaults are reported as considered commonplace. In this way, unhindered access to internet pornography now fills a 'sex education' vacuum for many adolescents (and adults) that is emotionally harmful and destructive to their relationships. Again, the saturation and limitless spread of 'knowledge' about human behaviour in an unregulated marketplace presents problems for what should be considered legitimately trustworthy. If the family, community, and schools are no longer the sole sources of knowledge and the moral guarantors for young people, their world is increasingly porous at time of intense vulnerability.

Help-seeking for emotional and psychological problems

A US review of national datasets revealed a worsening trend in student mental health over the last decade in which more than 41% screened positive for depression and 34% screened positive for anxiety in 2017–2018 (Downs & Eisenberg, 2012). Global student mental health surveys are similarly concerning (Bruffaerts et al., 2019). However, as also noted in the United Kingdom, there appear to be much lower levels of treatment than might have been expected for the prevalence of disorders. For example, among US college students with 12-month mental disorders, only 18% used mental health services (Blanco et al., 2008). Another US study found only 51% of students with suicidal ideation received any treatment (Duffy et al., 2019). In the United Kingdom, various major studies indicate that such high levels of unmet need may be a problem globally. What should be of serious concern to health services and government is that among the young people with a diagnosable mental illness, only one-third of these ever receive professional help (Green et al., 2005; World Federation for Mental Health, 2009). Even those with severe problems avoid seeking help or have considerable delays in getting appropriate help (Biddle et al., 2006; Burns et al., 1995; Goodman et al., 2002).

While timely detection and prediction of distress and sensitive intervention is crucial to reducing poor outcomes, academic institutions are poorly equipped to accurately detect and appropriately intervene when ordinary stressors begin to transition into problems of clinical seriousness. Thus, psychological distress tends to occur at times of reduced ability to deal with life pressures, exams, financial problems, and relationship break-up; all highly prevalent issues in the lives of young people. Limited institutional detection is exacerbated by low help-seeking among young people, due to stigma or poor emotional literacy.

Thus, evidence in the United Kingdom suggests that relatively few young men consult their GP prior to suicide (Appleby et al., 1996). According to various estimates, most (75%) adult psychiatric disorders have made an appearance before the age of 24 years, which means that a considerable level of psychiatric morbidity will have proceeded, perhaps deepened, undetected, and untreated. At first, one might consider that many of these cases are likely to have been mild, making little impact on the individual, but it also true that many others produce significant personal, social, and economic costs in terms of lost educational and employment opportunities, and high vulnerability to the criminal justice system. Additionally, there are potential health impacts; poor mental health is also associated with pathogenic lifestyles – eating disorders, obesity, sexual promiscuity, alcohol, and substance misuse – again, with negative life-course consequences. Adolescent risk-taking behaviours in themselves can be a maladaptive way of coping with emotional difficulties, once adopted tends to be carried into adult life.

There are several competing, sometimes intersecting, explanations for the gap between uptake of services and the prevalence of psychological distress. First, the individual's problems must be recognised and appropriately interpreted – the experience of distress and commensurate level of daily functioning may not reach a state that prompts the individual to seek help and/or sufficiently visible to family members to prompt them to obtain help. It may be that the problem is misrecognised and attributed to other phenomena – for example, parental downplaying distress as an adolescent phase, normal worries, bad behaviour. In some communities, behaviours may be perceived through a particular cultural lens – a religious problem or signs of supernatural forces. Second, psychological services must be available and accessible to adolescents with psychological problems, and a myriad of factors may be barriers here. Geographical location may limit availability and access. Thus, remote, and rural regions within most countries are often poorly served by health services of any kind, while financial constraints may prohibit the family's ability to travel in search of support. Family finance may also dictate the level and the quality of psychological services that they can access. In most Western countries, psychological therapies are available privately, not publicly funded, or free at the point of delivery. Language barriers and service knowledge may also be problem for many refugees and recently arrived migrant families.

Moreover, there are observable social class attitudinal differences to authority and the negotiation of needs and wishes with authority figures. Generally, children from the professional middle-classes tend to have a better understanding of the 'rules of the game' than children from disadvantaged and non-professional families (Lareau, 2015). If 'the game' and the 'rules' are controlled by those with socio-economic advantage, there are considerable disadvantages, including poor health outcomes, for those who don't know or can't conform to the social rules. Additionally, the collective experience of socio-economic disadvantage may lead to a lower sense of agency and control over one's own experiences but also drives a collective sense of mistrust and/or powerlessness (Whitehead et al., 2016).

Across all such difficulties, stigma plays a vital part. For some communities, the strength, depth, and impact of public stigma related to mental illness is more problematic for those who need help and here the question of what is at stake becomes a major deterrent to obtaining it. From an intersectional perspective, poverty, poor education, and ethnicity may drive some families into misrecognition, underplaying a mental health problem or denying that the problem exists, delaying seeking help, or searching for help that is inappropriate. The beliefs and attitudes of young people add to this complexity.

Mental health, trust, and help-seeking – adolescent perspectives

In a study on the mental health of minority ethnic pupils living in London (Leavey et al., 2004) we asked a deliberately vague, open-ended question 'what would you find helpful?' at the end of the questionnaire. Rather poignantly, many of those who scored highly as having psychological problems, and indeed many who didn't, replied that they 'wished that they had someone to talk to'. These words speak of disconnection, fear, loneliness and potentially, mistrust. In later studies we examined help-seeking and trust among adolescents. In a study among schoolchildren in North London we found that most of the participants preferred to speak with a parent, most commonly a mother, or their friends, if they experienced various emotional or psychological problems. Alarmingly, the preferences for contacting a family doctor were less than 30% and this was for 'hearing voices'. Teachers and school counsellors were rated even more poorly. Bearing in mind that these were posed as hypothetical situations, the idea that adolescents might be readily willing to consult with their friendship groups about mental health problems is perhaps stretching credulity and while young people often lack power in many help-seeking decisions, their responses do point to an antipathy towards health professionals, and perhaps professionals, generally. In this and later studies, focus group discussions revealed many of the key factors that influence young people's trust in family doctors and other health professionals.

As gatekeepers, general practitioners are well positioned to detect mental health problems in children and young people and to motivate parents to obtain care when needed (Zwaanswijk et al., 2003). While most young people attend general practice at least once a year (Elliott & Larson, 2004; Potts et al., 2001), these consultations are predominantly for physical conditions, mainly respiratory or dermatological (Potts et al., 2001). Help for more sensitive issues is sought from friends, family, or a trusted adult (Booth et al., 2004; Donald et al., 2000; Rickwood et al., 2007). In most cases the decision to seek professional help is usually made by a parent or other significant adults around the young person (Tylee et al., 2007). By the time they have reached adolescence, most young people's contact with a doctor will have almost certainly been for minor physical illnesses, but rarely for emotional problems. The emergence of psychological problems such as anxiety and depression are always troubling, regardless of age, but their arrival in youth can provoke a crisis of understanding as to what the symptoms mean, what (or who) has caused them, and when or if they will ever leave. Lacking the experience of being able to cope and 'push through' such problems, they can appear catastrophic, sometimes an existential threat, just at a time when personal and sexual relationships are beginning to form and one's sense of self has not been fully realised. It is not surprising then that a major chasm has appeared between the anticipation or idealisation of youth as a glorious time of hedonistic freedom and the sense of deflation of shame and despair experienced by many adolescents.

Families and subcultures of trust

The notion of adolescent independence may be more prevalent in some communities compared to others – the belief that one's children need to learn to fend for themselves 'to stand on their own two feet' – although commonly thought of as a (sub)cultural issue, the drive for adolescent independence is often a matter of financial resources and burden. Some parents may encourage and develop a milieu in which trusting others and shared decision-making is sensible and helpful. Children growing up in these environments may have less resistance to problem disclosure. Other children as we have suggested, develop a disposition towards maladaptive self-defence strategies which discourage talking about problems to 'strangers', or talking about problems at all. Unsurprisingly, there is an intergenerational transmission of suspicion and mistrust towards others through parents who are themselves emotionally remote and unavailable to their children, in many cases due to their own mental health problems.

Cultural issues related to social class may also play a role in children's trust and confidence to seek help outside the family. Various studies suggest that adolescents are more likely to trust their friends if they were to experience mental health problems. However, the evidence here is limited as these preferences are expressed in a hypothetical scenario. One can assume that not all friends are given the same level of trust and that in the event of a crisis, various psychological barriers may arise to prevent disclosure to friends. Moreover, depending on the level of visibility and functioning – distress and ability to go to school, among other things – the cues of vulnerability and protection will be acted upon by a responsible adult, who will then ascertain professional advice or more interventionist services. Importantly, the expansion of friendships in adolescence along is accompanied by intense social competition for group approval, influence, popularity, and leadership – and in evolutionary terms, sexual and reproductive success(Raihani & Bell, 2019). However, such competition also brings increased sensitivity to social threats and self-protection strategies that can also be harmful.

Health professionals and trust

The family doctor is generally the first professional health contact when a problem is noted. Importantly, various studies suggest that young people tend not to view their family doctor as trustworthy when asked if they would contact them in event of experiencing emotional or psychological problems. Our surveys showed that less than 30% of young people would not contact a GP if they had a mental health problem. Alongside the help-seeking surveys, we also ran a series of focus groups in London and Belfast to explore young people's trust in their family doctor. With rather alarming clarity, young people regarded the family doctor with a mixture of antipathy and frustration. The average GP could not be trusted. The sources of this distrust in mental health matters can be categorised as concerns related to personal privacy and fear of disclosure; uncertainty about rights, roles and responsibilities; service access problems. All relate strongly to vulnerability. First, young people lacked knowledge and information about the GP's role in relation to mental health, it was commonly assumed that family doctors only treated physical health problems. Additionally, across many of the groups, the participants were unsure if they were entitled to see the doctor without being accompanied by a parent. In fact, they had a right to consult a doctor autonomously. However, those who had made their own appointment were met with something akin to the inquisition (as the young people described it). Second, in relation to privacy, the participants felt extremely exposed as they considered discussing their problems with the GP.

> Once I tried to go to the GP on my own and when I went in she asked me where's my mum was and I told her - well I didn't go all by myself, my mum was waiting outside, but I went into the room on my own and she asked me where my mum was and I told her she was outside and she asked me why I came alone, and I thought - I didn't know what to say.... I just had the sort of feeling that I wanted to go on my own. I just ....there wasn't much that I needed to say to her but I just wanted to go on my own and she kept asking me why do you want to come on your own and stuff like that? And like (Classmate) said about the family thing, my GP is a family doctor as well and she asks a lot about oh you know what's happening about this and sort of relationship things and sort of gossip and things, and I don't like that because GPs shouldn't do that.
>
> (Hornsey girl)

This young person was obviously annoyed by the doctor's perceived refusal to regard her as having agency, and although we can assume that the GP was not being inquisitive about her family life out of idle curiosity, the girl experienced her questioning as intrusive, venturing beyond the acceptable boundaries of what a GP should ask. It is interesting that the GP's line of enquiry is regarded as gossip because this perception is the most likely source of anxiety and mistrust. Many of the young people make similar points that the GP is too close to their parents and would not observe patient confidentiality. Patient-doctor relationships are also clearly important. Commonly emphasised by young people are the doctors' personal qualities, the extent to which the family doctor is seen as warm, open, trustworthy, empathic, and able to engage with young people in ways that are considered as non-patronising. However, intergenerational differences may be difficult to tackle. The perception of many young people was that GPs were too old, and incapable of understanding their needs. Why would they discuss anything of importance with older people with whom they were unrelated? Additionally problematic for trust-building with medical professionals, is the lack of continuity in professional care, the difficulty in maintaining a relationship with a single clinician over several years. It is an issue not solely relevant to young people but perhaps more heightened because of the power imbalance. That is, given that young people feel that it requires considerable courage to contact the doctor and expose one's fears and anxieties, something that they may do incrementally, it feels unbearable that this may have to be repeated to different doctors at each visit. As highlighted by this exchange among young males in London.

> I just don't like telling people about my problems, like if I don't know them well and I don't really know my GP that well.
>
> (Interviewer)…Is that true for everybody else?
>
> (All agree)
>
> M… like, with my doctors there's not always the same doctor there's loads of different ones - I don't even know the name of them
>
> I also like the doctors 'cos they're friendly, but it's not always the same doctor, like whenever I go it's a different person, I don't know them so, it's always different so it's not like really too confidential.

Other service-related factors were also noted, such as 'front-desk' staff who were considered as intrusively and loudly inquisitive, and consultation times that were not appropriate to the lives of teenagers. A thread running through most of these discussions was a high degree of hypervigilance about being seen by one's peers as requiring any kind of help and at times, their discussions appeared to weave in and out of their concerns about relationships and sexuality, underscoring the criticism that services for young people, perhaps for all age groups, that our medical systems are overly compartmentalised. The lack of holistic approaches in adolescent health may undermine trust in medical care and are ultimately inefficient.

Continuity of care and trust

It was scary, I have to admit it was scary... ...I just didn't feel very sure about it because I was scared in case I had to go in and talk to him about everything over and over again – (remove the bandage from) old wounds and let them all out.

Challenges to the continuity of care and trust-building with health professionals are equally important to the provision of specialist mental health services for young people. Over the past decade or so, we have come to realise that there are key transition points in the structure of health service provision in most modern healthcare systems, commonly based on patient age, which can be experienced by the patient as a rupture. To lend an additional stress to this point, 18 is a critical transition time for various personal and social dimensions such as forming sexual relationships and making educational and employment choices.

In the United Kingdom, mental health services are organised based on Child and Adolescent Mental Health Services, usually provided up to the age of 18, and then Adult Mental Health Services and into Old Age Psychiatry (for people 65 years plus), and these tend to predominantly for people living with dementia and other neurological problems). The differences between youth and adult services are often over-drawn, but are nevertheless important in the culture, ethos, and delivery. In child and adolescent services, clinicians are often reluctant to provide a diagnosis – that it not to say they tolerate a great deal of diagnostic uncertainty but may consider a diagnostic label to be unhelpful at this early stage in the person's life. Importantly too, such clinicians are more likely to use systemic and psychotherapeutic approaches to treatment and management, largely absent in adult services. Thus, family members actively engaged in treatment and decision-making processes in adolescent services, tend to be excluded in adult care, where designated responsibility sits with the individual. This demarcation of roles and responsibilities may seem sensible. After all, in various areas of life that adult agency is assumed at 18 years (or younger) including the legal right to drink alcohol, driving a car, or getting married. However, many young people experience the move to adult mental health services as a painful and dramatic break – akin to 'falling off a cliff' as described to me.

You felt like you were getting pushed aside because you're not well or you're getting put to someone else, and you feel like that was too much to deal with. You're talking to someone about the way you feel, you're seeing your psychiatrist about your medication and then they're saying, 'we need to transfer you over' and it was just the whole impact of me talking to them about quite a lot of stuff and then they're like, 'we need to stop the brakes here and get you transferred over', sort of putting me on hold.

Crucial to young people was the kind of relationships with clinical staff. The aspects that they and their parents valued most about the service were it was trustworthy, accessible, available, and responsive. Again, as with the young participants in the schools study, confidentiality was underlined as pivotal to trust-building.

> I think it's good because -, it's confidential, you just know you can tell them anything, and even though there was some stuff that took me a while to say to them because it was so difficult to talk about, I still told them because they were very trustworthy people, and I knew it would help if I told them. And it did help.
>
> (Lisa, Service User)

> Just being able to talk to somebody and know that it's not going to go anywhere else. It's there in a file and it's locked away. Being able to trust somebody, it's just easier.
>
> (Christine, Service User)

While these young patients acknowledged that aspects of treatment must be shared with parents and carers, they also expected confidentiality in other issues. When confidentiality was perceived as breeched, without justification, patient-practitioner engagement was undermined and the therapeutic relationship damaged. One person described how he refused to continue seeing a psychiatrist when she *'broke his confidentiality twice'* by relaying information to his parents. In the quote below, another participant accepted the limitations of confidentiality, but regarded this line as crossed when her counsellor shared information with her social worker. It undermined the trust with her key worker and did not help an already faltering relationship:

> I think that's what didn't really help it. Because you were going in there trying to trust and build a rapport with that person, but maybe there are things that you're talking about that you don't want shared round with everybody. There's things that need to be disclosed and there's things that are not necessary but then if they're all coming in together, then things get shared that maybe shouldn't.
>
> (Belle, Service User)

The experience of 'being listened to' determined how young people assessed the quality of the relationship with practitioners and whether it could be described as *'real'* or authentic which young people sought to distinguish from the 'display' of caring. Real care involved a personal connection, the willingness to *'go the extra mile'*, being accessible and available, respecting and meeting the person where they are at. Importantly, as the comments of the young woman below suggest, the professional's motivation for caring is scrutinised. Thus, 'professional caring' is recognised as part of the professional's paid job, but not necessarily an emotional aspect of the patient-clinician relationship.

> They were real, they weren't all this bullshit, hugging and... []. Like, they weren't fake, and you could tell they actually cared, because the one thing I

said from the start, and I would have said this to them quite regularly, I was like 'Why do you care?' and they'd be like 'We do care', and I'm like, 'No, you get paid to care. There's a difference.' And they were like 'No, we do care.' And I'm like 'No, you get paid to care'. But these two actually cared and I just knew that. And they were real with me. They weren't fake, they weren't sticking to the book.

(Fiona, Service User)

Ideally, as young people in adolescent psychiatric services approach the transition to adult psychiatric services, arrangements such as a period of parallel care and joint working with AMHS clinicians, will have been instigated, so that the young patient can gradually get to know and trust the new clinicians. Unfortunately, this process of familiarisation and continuity tends to be exceptional. This means that at the peak age for onset when continuity and trust are crucial, the healthcare system may be failing many young patients.

In summary, adolescence is a critical developmental period in which young people are obliged to adapt to significant physiological and psychological changes that many struggle to integrate. For such children, these changes profoundly impact not just their relationship with others but also their self-relationship creating a sense of estrangement and being lost. However, feelings of bewilderment and anxiety are accompanied by intense feelings of shame, of 'being seen' by others who may harm them in some way.

Notes

1 While previous generations had anxieties about television and adolescent health, evidence suggests that television watching has much less negative impact.
2 Similar to the positives and negative aspects of motor car use, this will always be an impossible issue due to the imprecision of the question.

References

Appleby, L., Amos, T., Doyle, U., Tomenson, B., & Woodman, M. (1996). General practitioners and young suicides: A preventive role for primary care. *The British Journal of Psychiatry, 168*(3), 330–333. https://doi.org/10.1192/bjp.168.3.330

Biddle, L., Donovan, J., Gunnell, D., & Sharp, D. (2006). Young adults' perceptions of GPs as a help source for mental distress: A qualitative study. *British Journal of General Practice, 56*, 924–931.

Blanco, C., Okuda, M., Wright, C., Hasin, D. S., Grant, B. F., Liu, S. M., & Olfson, M. (2008). Mental health of college students and their non-college-attending peers: Results from the National Epidemiologic Study on alcohol and related conditions. *Archives of General Psychiatry, 65*(12), 1429–1437. https://doi.org/10.1001/archpsyc.65.12.1429

Booth, M. L., Bernard, D., Quine, S., Kang, M. S., Usherwood, T., Alperstein, G., & Bennett, D. L. (2004). Access to health care among Australian adolescents young people's perspectives and their sociodemographic distribution. *Journal of Adolescent Health, 34*(1), 97–103. https://doi.org/10.1016/j.jadohealth.2003.06.011

Brailovskaia, J., Swarlik, V. J., Grethe, G. A., Schillack, H., & Margraf, J. (2022). Experimental longitudinal evidence for causal role of social media use and physical activity in COVID-19 burden and mental health. *Z Gesundh Wiss*, 1–14. https://doi.org/10.1007/s10389-022-01751-x

Bridges, A. J., & Morokoff, P. J. (2011). Sexual media use and relational satisfaction in heterosexual couples. *Personal Relationships*, *18*(4), 562–585.

Bruffaerts, R., Mortier, P., Auerbach, R. P., Alonso, J., Hermosillo De la Torre, A. E., Cuijpers, P., Demyttenaere, K., Ebert, D. D., Green, J. G., Hasking, P., Stein, D. J., Ennis, E., Nock, M. K., Pinder-Amaker, S., Sampson, N. A., Vilagut, G., Zaslavsky, A. M., & Kessler, R. C. (2019). Lifetime and 12-month treatment for mental disorders and suicidal thoughts and behaviors among first year college students. *International Journal of Methods in Psychiatric Research*, *28*(2), e1764. https://doi.org/10.1002/mpr.1764

Burns, B. J., Costello, E. J., Angold, A., Tweed, D., Stangl, D., Farmer, E. M., & Erkanli, A. (1995). Children's mental health service use across service sectors. *Health Affairs*, *14*(3), 147–159. https://doi.org/10.1377/hlthaff.14.3.147

Donald, M., Dower, J., Lucke, J., & Raphael, B. (2000). *The Queensland Young Peoples' Mental Health Survey Report*.

Downs, M. F., & Eisenberg, D. (2012). Help seeking and treatment use among suicidal college students. *Journal of American College Health*, *60*(2), 104–114. https://doi.org/10.1080/07448481.2011.619611

Duffy, M. E., Twenge, J. M., & Joiner, T. E. (2019). Trends in mood and anxiety symptoms and suicide-related outcomes among U.S. Undergraduates, 2007-2018: Evidence from two national surveys. *Journal of Adolescent Health*, *65*(5), 590–598. https://doi.org/10.1016/j.jadohealth.2019.04.033

Elliott, B., & Larson, J. (2004). Adolescents in mid-sized and rural communities: Foregone care, perceived barriers, and risk factors. *Journal of Adolescent Health*, *35*, 303–309.

Goodman, R., Ford, T., & Meltzer, H. (2002). Mental health problems of children in the community: 18 month follow up. *BMJ*, *324*(7352), 1496–1497. http://bmj.com

Green, H., McGinnity, Á, Meltzer, H., Ford, T., & Goodman, R. H. (2005). *Mental Health of Children and Young People in Britain, 2004*.

Lareau, A. (2015). Cultural knowledge and social inequality. *American Sociological Review*, *80*(1), 1–27.

Leavey, G., Hollins, K., King, M., Papadopoulos, C., & Barnes, J. (2004). Psychological disorder amongst refugee and migrant children in London. *Social Psychiatry & Psychiatric Epidemiology*, *39*, 191–195.

Leavey, G., Rosato, M., Harding, S., Corry, D., Divin, N., & Breslin, G. (2020). Adolescent mental health problems, suicidality and seeking help from general practice: A cross-sectional study (Northern Ireland Schools and Wellbeing study). *Journal of Affective Disorders*, *274*, 535–544. https://doi.org/10.1016/j.jad.2020.05.083

Lin, L. Y., Sidani, J. E., Shensa, A., Radovic, A., Miller, E., Colditz, J. B., Hoffman, B. L., Giles, L. M., & Primack, B. A. (2016). Association between social media use and depression among U.S. young adults. *Depress Anxiety*, *33*(4), 323–331. https://doi.org/10.1002/da.22466

Marchant, A., Hawton, K., Stewart, A., Montgomery, P., Singaravelu, V., Lloyd, K., Purdy, N., Daine, K., & John, A. (2018). Correction: A systematic review of the relationship between internet use, self-harm and suicidal behaviour in young people: The good, the bad and the unknown. *PLOS One*, *13*(3), e0193937. https://doi.org/10.1371/journal.pone.0193937

Marino, C., Gini, G., Vieno, A., & Spada, M. M. (2018). The associations between problematic Facebook use, psychological distress and well-being among adolescents and young adults: A systematic review and meta-analysis. *Journal of Affective Disorders*, *226*, 274–281. https://doi.org/10.1016/j.jad.2017.10.007

Newlove-Delgado, T., Marcheselli, F., Williams, T., Mandalia, D., Davis, J., McManus, S., Savic, M., Treloar, W., & Ford, T. (2022). *Mental health of children and young people in England, 2022.*

Potts, Y., Gillies, M., & Wood, S. (2001). Lack of mental well-being in 15-year-olds: An undisclosed iceberg? *Family Practice, 18*(1), 95–100.

Purba, A. K., Thomson, R. M., Henery, P. M., Pearce, A., Henderson, M., & Katikireddi, S. V. (2023). Social media use and health risk behaviours in young people: Systematic review and meta-analysis. *BMJ, 383*, e073552. https://doi.org/10.1136/bmj-2022-073552

Raihani, N. J., & Bell, V. (2019). An evolutionary perspective on paranoia. *Nature Human Behavior, 3*(2), 114–121. https://doi.org/10.1038/s41562-018-0495-0

Reyna, V. F., Estrada, S. M., DeMarinis, J. A., Myers, R. M., Stanisz, J. M., & Mills, B. A. (2011). Neurobiological and memory models of risky decision making in adolescents versus young adults. *Journal of Experimental Psychology: Learning, Memory, and Cognition, 37*(5), 1125–1142. https://doi.org/10.1037/a0023943

Reyna, V. F., & Farley, F. (2006). Risk and rationality in adolescent decision making: Implications for theory, practice, and public policy. *Psychological Science in the Public Interest, 7*(1), 1–44. https://doi.org/10.1111/j.1529-1006.2006.00026.x

Richter, D., Wall, A., Bruen, A., & Whittington, R. (2019). Is the global prevalence rate of adult mental illness increasing? Systematic review and meta-analysis. *Acta Psychiatrica Scandinavica, 140*(5), 393–407. https://doi.org/10.1111/acps.13083

Rickwood, D. J., Deane, F. P., & Wilson, C. J. (2007). *When and how do young people seek professional help for mental health problems?* Retrieved September 2010 from http://www.mja.com.au/public/issues/187_07_011007/ric10279_fm.html

Riehm, K. E., Feder, K. A., Tormohlen, K. N., Crum, R. M., Young, A. S., Green, K. M., Pacek, L. R., La Flair, L. N., & Mojtabai, R. (2019). Associations between time spent using social media and internalizing and externalizing problems among US youth. *JAMA Psychiatry, 76*(12), 1266–1273. https://doi.org/10.1001/jamapsychiatry.2019.2325

Sedgwick, R., Epstein, S., Dutta, R., & Ougrin, D. (2019). Social media, internet use and suicide attempts in adolescents. *Current Opinion in Psychiatry, 32*(6), 534–541. https://doi.org/10.1097/yco.0000000000000547

Shensa, A., Escobar-Viera, C. G., Sidani, J. E., Bowman, N. D., Marshal, M. P., & Primack, B. A. (2017). Problematic social media use and depressive symptoms among U.S. Young adults: A nationally-representative study. *Social Science & Medicine, 182*, 150–157. https://doi.org/10.1016/j.socscimed.2017.03.061

Stewart, D. N., & Szymanski, D. M. (2012). Young adult Women's reports of their male romantic Partner's pornography use as a correlate of their self-esteem, relationship quality, and sexual satisfaction. *Sex Roles, 67*(5), 257–271. https://doi.org/10.1007/s11199-012-0164-0

Teppers, E., Luyckx, K., Klimstra, T. A., & Goossens, L. (2014). Loneliness and Facebook motives in adolescence: A longitudinal inquiry into directionality of effect. *Journal of Adolescence, 37*(5), 691–699. https://doi.org/10.1016/j.adolescence.2013.11.003

Thomas, R., Sanders, S., Doust, J., Beller, E., & Glasziou, P. (2015). Prevalence of attention-deficit/hyperactivity disorder: A systematic review and meta-analysis. *Pediatrics, 135*(4), e994–1001. https://doi.org/10.1542/peds.2014-3482

Tromholt, M. (2016). The Facebook experiment: Quitting Facebook leads to higher levels of well-being. *Cyberpsychology, Behavior, and Social Networking, 19*(11), 661–666. https://doi.org/10.1089/cyber.2016.0259

Tylee, A., Haller, D. M., Graham, T., Churchill, R., & Sanci, L. A. (2007). Youth-friendly primary-care services: How are we doing and what more needs to be done? *The Lancet, 369*(9572), 1565–1573. https://doi.org/10.1016/S0140-6736(07)60371-7

Whitehead, M., Pennington, A., Orton, L., Nayak, S., Petticrew, M., Sowden, A., & White, M. (2016). How could differences in 'control over destiny' lead to socio-economic inequalities in health? A synthesis of theories and pathways in the living environment. *Health Place*, *39*, 51–61. https://doi.org/10.1016/j.healthplace.2016.02.002

Willoughby, B. J., Carroll, J. S., Busby, D. M., & Brown, C. C. (2016). Differences in pornography use among couples: Associations with satisfaction, stability, and relationship processes. *Archives of Sexual Behavior*, *45*, 145–158.

World Federation for Mental Health. (2009). *Mental Health in Primary Care: Enhancing Treatment and Promoting Mental Health*. World Federation for Mental Health. Retrieved May 2010 from http://www.wfmh.org/00WorldMentalHealthDay.htm

Wright, P. J., Tokunaga, R. S., Kraus, A., & Klann, E. (2017). Pornography consumption and satisfaction: A meta-analysis. *Human Communication Research*, *43*(3), 315–343.

Zwaanswijk, M., Verhaak, P. F. M., Bensing, J. M., van der Ende, J., & Verhulst, F. C. (2003). Help seeking for emotional and behavioural problems in children and adolescents. *European Child & Adolescent Psychiatry*, *12*(4), 153–161. http://dx.doi.org/10.1007/s00787-003-0322-6

Chapter 6

Trust and Mistrust in Healthcare

Although trust is often described as a pivotal characteristic in medical relationships it has received relatively little attention in health research, compared to the role of trust in political systems or business, for example. It is also generally absent as a measure in health outcomes research, even in studies of patient satisfaction with hospital care and treatment; a striking omission given the multidimensional nature and role of trust in confidentiality, communication, and decision-making, indeed almost every dimension of medical care (Pearson & Raeke, 2000). Trust plays an essential role in the very fundamental processes and outcomes of sickness and healing in which sickness defined as the biological and behavioural expressions of disease and injury (regardless of medical tradition, and healing as the 'culturally meaningful social responses aimed at undoing or preventing the effects of disease and injury' (Fabrega, 1997, p. iv).

Western 'scientific' medicine has developed over the past several hundred years to become the dominant global form of healing, in part because of the West's political, economic, and technological power institutionalised through huge private and public investment in research and development and the flow of evidence that underpin and promote this dominance. Porter argues that throughout human history most peoples and cultures have situated and understood life events and stages – birth, death, health, and suffering – in relationship to the wider cosmos and everything contained within it, all external phenomena both natural and supernatural. Western culture increasingly focussed on the individual and a preoccupation with the self – in Gidden's terms the 'project of the self' which has scant regard for the significance of the external unless as signifiers of an 'alternative' spirituality, or what Bourdieu might regard as a distinguishing expression of cultural capital. Over centuries Western medicine began to look away from elements of the cosmos to focus more resolutely and intensely on sickness as expressed by the individual human body and what is passed between bodies, human and non-human. As industrialisation and urbanisation developed, so too did the scope of medicine as it gradually and begrudgingly recognised the origins of disease (and disorder) in the social body. In late industrial societies medicine had been co-opted into the coterminous needs and demands of the state and industrial companies. The medical gaze widened beyond the individual anatomy to acknowledge the social

DOI: 10.4324/9781003326687-6

dimensions of disease. Well-functioning productive industries and economies depended on well-functioning productive labour, and healthy economies demand healthy citizens to produce wealth and fight wars in an increasingly competitive world.

Although the COVID-19 pandemic revealed the integral connections between medicine, economics, and politics, these relationships had been cemented more than a century before. With enormous authority and reach, medicine demonstrated its influence, touching upon and dictating the negotiation of every aspect of human activity. While politicians call the shots, physicians often pulled the strings. Medicine had been transformed during the 20th century from a set of loose uncoordinated and unregulated practices undertaken by disparate, usually self-employed practitioners into a complex purpose-driven and designed institution, supported by bureaucratic structures. The 'medical machine' as Porter describes it, had 'a programme dedicated to the investigation of all that is objective and measurable and to the pursuit of high-tech, closely monitored practice. It has acquired extraordinary momentum' (Porter, 1997, p. 629). Nevertheless, the triumph of Western medicine is often contested and arguably difficult to assess. The average lifespan in Western societies has been extended by tens of years but much of the gains in mortality can be explained by lifting people out of absolute poverty, improvements in housing and education, and public health measures in sanitation and diet. While there are extraordinary medical breakthroughs in the treatment of cancer, organ transplant, genetic engineering, and vaccinations, these triumphs are overshadowed and undone by human self-harm wrought by environmental pollution, climate change ecological disasters, and obesogenic diseases emerging from the food industry.

Those who most conspicuously represent healthcare are the frontline clinical staff, the doctors and nurses, who have come to symbolise human virtue – kindness, love, compassion, patience. With some exceptions, doctors and nurses are firmly embedded as a benign presence in Western cultural narratives, assuming an intimate familiarity in collective consciousness. Thus, akin to family members, hospital staff are almost universally regarded by the public with high, possibly idealised, levels of trust. However, a cursory examination of the literature on trust and healthcare refers to doctors despite the fact that most patient contact in hospitals is likely to be with nursing and auxiliary staff. That aside, patients trust doctors because they are highly trained professionals, deriving authority from patients' acknowledgement of this (Friedson, 1960). Much of the discussion of trust characterises it as a type of blind faith (Barbalet, 2009; Giddens, 1991) an unconscious assumption that expectations will be met in situations of vulnerability, implicitly any degree of intentionality on the part of the trustor. While a significant proportion of moment-to-moment human behaviour has an unconscious appearance, action is based on an intentionality towards a future outcome. Intentionality is underpinned by a belief that to achieve this or that outcome particular actions and conditions must be met. In the sense that beliefs are associated with an anticipated outcome, we can regard beliefs an inhabiting a closely overlapping cognitive framework with trust. Like trust, beliefs are contingent and lacking in factual certainty.

Jens Rydgren offers a definition of beliefs as often unconsciously developed 'propositions about the world in which a person is at least confident' (2012, p. 77). He also outlines several principle processes of belief-formation that are also recognisable as those in trust-formation. Thus, beliefs develop in some combination of direct observation, information received from external sources including those provided through socialisation; inferential evidence derived but beyond observation; and beliefs that are adapted to fit desires or as mechanisms to reduce dissonance. Individuals may be predisposed to optimism and trust because they have been socialised to believe that this is ethically or strategically important or, to adopt a trusting stance that is aligned with beliefs and actions. Human beings seek information and explanation for phenomena, more usually an understanding directed towards problems and misfortune, including system failures and poor health. Striving towards 'cognitive closure', failure to comprehend past significant events, or what is likely to occur, tend to provoke anxiety, discomfort, and conflict. To mitigate against such stressors, individuals situate such events within an explanatory model or belief framework even if, as they often are, not entirely coherent or consistent.

While beliefs may underpin intentional action, they do not necessarily emerge from conscious processes. Similar to the formation and use of stereotypes, beliefs as cognitive strategies operate within a ready-made cultural repertoire, used when a situation requires a response, and maintained until their validity or desirability is questioned and/or provokes cognitive dissonance (Hart et al., 2009). Accepting that social approval and trust in clinicians and other professionals are sometimes undermined by system failures or malign actions in healthcare organisations, breeches of trust are rapidly 'forgotten' by the general public and never result in widespread disaffection, partly explained by the limited alternatives in healthcare provision. Even in the United States patients may switch doctors, or even sue them, but they tend to maintain a loyalty to Western medicine overall rather than adopt other healing systems.

The management of trust in healthcare

It is assumed that clinicians, particularly those working in the public sector are, theoretically, unburdened by the influences and demands of market forces and therefore free to focus on the patient's best interests. However, few people outside those connected with the health sector, clinicians, academics, policy-makers, and managers, are aware of healthcare rationing and the economic pressures on clinical decision-making. Indeed, the actuality of healthcare rationing is seldom discussed or acknowledged. However, while the need for social goods such as healthcare maybe limitless, the availability of resources to meet these needs are finite, forcing difficult choices to enable a reasonably fair balance across all other social goods and the people who seek them. Individuals seeking healthcare may be denied a potentially beneficial treatment based on scarcity because there is always some level of risk that the patient may not benefit or that the benefit may not be sufficiently beneficial, years of extra life or quality of life, to justify the economic costs

(Scheunemann & White, 2011). While rationing guidelines are generally followed by most physicians, often enforced by management systems, there remains a high level of ambivalence about rigid enforcement. While many will accept the need for rationing health care services, they also seek to establish personal professional autonomy and judgement in doing so for particular services and patients (Strech et al., 2009). Willingness to assert agency in the face of growing bureaucratisation also produces personal risk in terms of job security but may be essential for personal integrity, especially in occupations characterised as vocational – employment that carries emotional commitment and appears to transcend financial reward.

Although trust may underpin the patient–doctor relationship, patients can never be sure that their expectations of optimal care can be met and are often unaware that decisions about treatment may have been made elsewhere by managers or arrived at arbitrarily. Moreover, in situations of extreme patient vulnerability in which there are no alternatives of care, it is somewhat implausible to characterise the patient's attitude or belief towards the physician as one of 'trust', and this bracketing of trust is more obviously demonstrated in the hospitalisation of patients in psychiatric emergencies. However, interest in trust in healthcare has emerged through a more general exploration of organisational culture and processes, the balancing of managerial mechanisms for monitoring and control of employees and outputs, and customer satisfaction and developing efficiencies. These interests in trust are added to the concerns within social sciences for understanding its role in the making and breaking of social stability, all emphasising the instrumental value of trust. In healthcare, trust matters across several key areas such as: (1) therapeutic engagement with patients; (2) the smooth uptake of public health messages and interventions such as vaccines, safe limits for alcohol use, and speed limits; (3) reducing internal friction within health system transactions; (4) improving inter-agency communication; (4) the protection of patient privacy; (5) mitigation of legal risks; (6) staff cooperation, commitment, and retention; and (7) staff esteem-building through patient trust.

Older corporate culture and organisational design appear to be overly reliant on rigid, hierarchical structures in which authority and command dominate the working culture but at the cost of producing low trust and obtaining staff engagement. Younger, more modern organisations see productive benefits within flatter structures, and a culture that emphasises solidarity, democratic processes in decision-making – all of which contribute to more satisfied and engaged staff, less prone to stress and burn-out, high staff sickness rates and turnover. What is being attempted in such organisations is a recreation of family-type solidarity, the members of which have a shared understanding of the goals, the commitment to achieving them, and a loyalty to the group. Trust in the goals and the organisation means that staff are more likely to give 'more of themselves' than they are contractually obliged, beneficial to the organisation perhaps but potentially exploitative and unhealthy to the employees. Despite shifts in progressive work culture and ethos, there has been a revitalisation of management practices that operate in low-trust, high-scrutiny organisations based on set target attainment and performance attainment. Managerialism may have marginal and short-term benefits in staff per-formance, producing high levels in conformity with processes but in rigidly bu-reaucratising staff–client (patient) engagement, there are considerable disbenefits created by removing informal interactions. Moreover, as we observed among the teaching profession, similarly conceptualised as a vocation, the continuous external scrutiny and assessment of practices is often damaging to professional autonomy, self-esteem, and detrimental to mental health (Skinner et al., 2021).

Healthcare in developed Western systems is seldom the responsibility of cli-nicians. Behind them is an intricate supply line of technicians, clerical officers, pharmacists, and so on, without whom, most treatment and care would fail. In this sense, trust is condensed and simplified through embodiment in the institutional representatives, the clinician. But what are the origins and justification for trust in healthcare; what are the determinants that underpin trust and what factors are likely to undermine it? Healthcare systems may aspire to create a similar ethos in which trust is at the centre of presenting a strong clinical team to the patient. As in other social situations, when trust breaks down, so does the delivery of the desired out-comes. Hospital patients particularly, are acutely aware when staff relationships are mistrustful and only grudgingly cooperative. Hospital settings are intimate places where patients can feel and absorb a considerable amount of information, visual, verbal and non-verbal, and difficult and inauthentic exchanges between staff are easily detected. In situations of staff conflict, vulnerable patients who need emo-tional containment can become anxious. Mistrust between staff transmitted to pa-tients may be transformed into an erosion of patients' confidence and trust in staff.

Trust – the placebo in healthcare

Recognising the 'whole person' behind a disease rather than as a disease entity – patients are still referred to as their disorder – has been a long-standing episte-mological and ethical concern in medicine, probably emerging from a professional demand for objectivity and the transfer of medical care from generalist medicine at the patient's home to specialist medicine in the hospital. The relentless expan-sion of digital technology in healthcare adds another level of objectification of the patient, creating more patient–clinician distance.

The importance of trust in reducing objectivity and clinical distance emerges from both its intrinsic and instrumental dimensions. It is commonly acknowledged as the basis of the patient–doctor relationship and its defining characteristic, hold-ing the same qualitative emotional significance found in other intimate relation-ships, love or friendship (Rhodes & Strain, 2000). Instrumentally, trust provides the basis for effective (and more efficient) therapeutic processes, facilitating help-seeking, adherence to treatment, and continuity of care. Sitting somewhere be-tween its intrinsic and instrumental values, it may be a bridge between mind–body interactions, associated with placebo effects in clinical outcomes. Placebo has been described as the 'total drug effect', but in the absence of a drug. While often disre-garded as a nuisance, the inert comparator in drug trials, science has become much more interested in the effects, psychological, physiological, or both, resulting from the belief of the patient (or the doctor).

Important placebo effects have been noted in studies of pain, depression, anxiety, insomnia, and Parkinson's disease (Benedetti et al., 2003). Importantly, while it was widely understood that the placebo effect was only possible when participants were 'tricked' into believing that they received a real treatment, other evidence suggested that the placebo could be introduced with an 'open label', that is even though the patients were not deceived, the effect remained (Kaptchuk et al., 2010). While we cannot fully understand the mechanisms that underpin placebo, it is likely to be a component of all healing modalities and most likely associated with expectancies – again, an optimistic (or in the case of nocebo, pessimistic) future-oriented anticipation of a good outcome. One theory suggests that the placebo effect is a learned response, through which various types of cues (verbal, conditioned, and social) activate expectancies producing placebo effects trough the central nervous system. In other words, a range of cues combine to generate central expectancies about treatment responses that drive the placebo effect regardless of cultural context (Colagiuri et al., 2015).

Contingent on the level of severity, the occurrence of sickness and injury places the individual in a state of dependency on others, from which emerges issues of trust, in systems, organisations, and individuals. At home and in the community where the preponderance of healthcare is provided, trust is predicated not just on the caregiver's competencies but on their desire to assist our health and care, whatever that takes. Trust in this context is highly interpersonal and based on past experience and knowledge about the caregiver's personality, among other characteristics. However, if trust is predicated on risk and vulnerability, this raises the conundrum of just how much vulnerability is present in this relationship before trust is considered no longer relevant; that is, an individual believes that his or her health condition is at such a critical point that no alternative options remain but to trust the caregiver, a *will* to trust, as it were – similarly, the absence of choice in the context of monopolistic healthcare. Here we have to distinguish between trusting attitudes and trusting behaviours, whereby the former is characterised by an optimism of treatment and acceptance of vulnerability – an optimism based perhaps on previous knowledge and experience within the healthcare system. For others, treatment may be approached with a resignation and pessimism resonant of mistrust (Hall et al., 2001). Therefore, trust in informal caregiving as well as medical care is constituted by having a positive attitude rather than the display of trusting behaviour alone.

Cognitive and emotional dimensions of trust

Luhmann (1988) distinguishes between *trust* and *confidence* the latter referring to a rational expectation based on previous experience or knowledge. Usually described as *cognitive-based trust*, patients require their clinicians to have competencies and skills that can be relied upon to achieve desired outcomes. In the absence of a long-term relationship with a physician, and this is increasingly rare, information about the physician's competence and reliability may be transmitted by other patients or as information provided by healthcare organisations. An individual physician may also obtain a reputation vicariously through their institutional affiliation. We might argue that these are formal and measurable aspects of care that contribute to trustworthiness of organisations and their employees, clinical and otherwise, such as qualifications and experience of staff, staffing levels, satisfaction with consultation and treatment times, positive patient outcomes, and so on. However, various less tangible and more subjective dimensions of trust sit within the patient's assessment of the clinician and the latter's ability to convey the qualities that constitute and increase the appearance of trustworthiness. Karen Cook and colleagues (2004) provide evidence about the determinants of patient–physician trust. Physician behaviours, specifically interactions with patients that convey an authentic concern for the person, rather than being treated as another 'case'. This kind of personal connection is conveyed by verbal and non-verbal behaviours that underpin a therapeutic alliance also assist in reducing the power asymmetry between patient and doctor, understood as a significant barrier to trust. In connecting emotionally with a patient's vulnerability, doctors may demonstrate not just empathy but a shared commitment to a good outcome.

One's early experiences of caregiving by others within a particular family milieu are likely to create the conditions for the individual's ability to trust over the life-course. The parental attachment style matters significantly, with disorganised attachment in childhood being a powerful predictor for severe psychopathology and maladjustment, and commonly associated with unresolved loss or trauma in the caregiver (Green & Goldwyn, 2002). However, even with more benign parenting, the informal caregiver may have a full-time occupation and may not have the time or has other interests which undermine the quality of caring. They may simply lack compassion or, after a while, find the role tedious. These and other similar factors undermine interpersonal trust, motivating the patient towards a state of self-dependency, again, depending on the level of severity. Once a doctor is required, the patient begins on a pathway into a system which, increasingly, is less knowable and unpredictable. Assuming that the familiar gentle family doctor is now only an object of historical interest, the patient's dependencies are now extended to a wide network of individuals, administrators, clinicians, laboratories, technical processes, and communication technology to which they have no direct contact. Healthcare in this respect is an institutional black box, highly abstract, requiring a different kind of trust but one offered symbolic 'humanised' form via doctors and nursing staff. They sit at the patient-facing end of healthcare, behind which is a complex web of people and processes, all containing a myriad of risks over which the patient has no control and little knowledge. At the front-end of healthcare, patients are often obliged to submit to requests from strangers, often in front of other strangers, that would otherwise be unthinkable in other circumstances – the recording of private, sometimes intimate information, removal of clothes and personal items, submission to needles and probes, share sleeping and toilet facilities with people unknown. The ability of clinicians to build patient trust facilitates a smoother treatment process, removing barriers to cooperation and engagement that may be a risk to good outcomes. Luhmann's (1988) view of familiarity as an important mechanism in the calculation of risk is appropriate in that trust-building and the mitigation of risk are more likely with clinicians with whom we have continuity of care. We also recognise 'familiarisation' as a strategy that individuals use in potentially violent situations whereby the victim provides the perpetrator with personal information life, that they have a family and so on, creating a subjective intimacy in the hope that this will reduce the risk of suffering.

Continuity of care

Relationships that are built over time are more likely to have the characteristics that constitute a 'thick' form of trust. While encapsulated within context of healthcare, such relationships can extend beyond this context but run the risk of provoking other problems related to conflict of interest, concerns of confidentiality and the potential for exploitation, sexual and financial impropriety, for example. For these reasons, most jurisdictions will have a mixture of guidelines and regulations on set parameters for physician–patient relationships, with sanctions for transgressions.

The concept of continuity of care is regarded as an ideal condition for trust-building, mostly based on long-term healthcare provision by the same physician or clinical team in the pursuit of seamless, coherent, and efficient care. However, to the chronological may be added other dimensions such as geographical, interdisciplinary, interpersonal, and informational. But is also the case that the study of continuity of care has expanded over recent years to accommodate variation in concepts and scope, that is, within and across organisations. At its most basic, continuity of care is generally interpreted as uninterrupted care by a clinician or clinical team. However, increasing numbers of people living longer with multiple and comorbid conditions and complex care needs including cognitive or functional impairment may require a range of health and social care services, and these are often fragmented and uncoordinated. The concept of patient-centred care meaning that the patient's needs take priority over the needs of the system and constituent parts, has also become woven into discussion of what continuity means.

Theoretically, better patient outcomes can be achieved by continuity of care compared to care provided by different people at different times over the patient's lifetime or at different points in episodes of care (Cabana & Jee, 2004). Thus, a mutuality of trust can be developed over time through an accumulation of knowledge about the patient, their needs, personality, social situation and support, and dispositions. The knowledge that may assist the doctor is not limited to biomedical facts but rather, can include understanding the patient's personhood – the totality of their social and spiritual needs and concerns, that is, what matters to them, and their support networks that may influence treatment and clinical decisions. However, trust-building potential is predicated on choice, the ability of patients to seek alternatives, which for some patients may not be possible, for financial reasons, or monopoly due to geographical limitations. Indeed, patients' desires to leave may be constrained by a desire not to offend the doctor or to be viewed as a 'bad' patient, a troublemaker.

There are national differences in patient freedom to choose doctors, and doctors rights to refuse patients. In the United Kingdom, doctors in primary care are limited in refusing or rejecting patients, compared to the flexibility in the United States (Schoen et al., 2004). Nevertheless, cross-national evidence suggests that while most physicians highly value continuity of care regardless of the funding system, they acknowledge its fragility – particularly in the United States where health insurance managed care creates more frequent patient switching of doctors, presumably to drive competition and squeeze costs. Managed care, however, has been criticised by mechanic and others due to its corrosive effects on the doctor–patient relationship by constraining the physician's freedom to make patient-centred choices based on personal needs. Time pressures in patient consultations, frequent discontinuities in care, and increased physician responsibilities in advocacy and care allocation, add to the deterioration in patient–physician trust (Mechanic, 1998).

Those most impacted by fragmented care are those with multiple morbidities. As noted previously, people with a severe mental illness such as schizophrenia die much younger than people without these disorders, as much as 20 years. They also have a much higher risk than people in the general population of having multiple comorbidities such as diabetes, coronary heart disease, stroke, and chronic kidney disease. For example, in our study of comorbidity and mortality we found that people with severe mental illness had a threefold risk of having three or more comorbidities compared to other patients, after considering various socioeconomic and other factors. Such patents were twice as likely to have kidney disease, chronic obstructive pulmonary disorder, and diabetes mellitus (McCarter et al., 2023). We also noted that people with severe mental illness, developed these life-limiting conditions at younger ages than other patients, despite our expectation of contact with specialist treatment at a later stage. There is considerable evidence that people with mental health problems are provided sub-optimal care, or at least, have sub-optimal contact with non-psychiatric healthcare services, for various reasons including low GP consultation rates, and under-recognition by primary care physicians and others. The concept of 'overshadowing" whereby the physical health problems of a patient with severe mental illness tend to be overlooked by clinicians whose 'gaze' is too firmly fixed on the psychiatric diagnosis. Thus, people with schizophrenia are less likely to be offered examination but also, may be less likely to accept treatment compared to non-psychiatric patients (Attar et al., 2017). As many people with schizophrenia are less likely to be married or in partnership, they also lack the encouragement and social support that helps maintain medical connections.[1]

What then is the basis of trust in healthcare and does this differ between social and cultural contexts? Generally, it is not about the clinicians' competencies, their knowledge, and skills; we can assume that 'genuine' doctors have undergone rigorous training and are appropriately qualified to practice in their particular speciality.[2] While these elements are associated with patient satisfaction and confidence with care, they don't in themselves equate to trust. In this aspect, we can add that while trustworthiness may overlap with trust, it is also clear that trust can easily be misplaced in some physicians and/or institutions. The extent to which trust can be assessed as either justified or not, tends to be normative rather than measurable, since the unpacking of trust attributes is a subjective exercise, and therefore variable. In some respects, there is potential for the patient's trust to sit uncomfortably balanced whereby a trusting and optimistic interpersonal (emotional) relationship is held with a clinician who has poor clinical skills or, conversely, mistrust can be directed towards a highly skilled clinician lacking warmth (Hall et al., 2001).

Doctors, nurses, and other healthcare staff possess considerably high levels of public and patient esteem and trust, compared to other public servants. Although the enormous public acclaim that healthcare staff in the United Kingdom and elsewhere received during the COVID-19 pandemic was somewhat ephemeral, as a profession they are nevertheless idealised by patients, possessing virtues that cannot, of course, be fully realised in the course of clinical practice and hospital routines. For patients facing life-threatening health problems, an exaggerated sense of optimism (hope) and trust in physicians may be understandable and be salutogenic through a placebo effect but also heightens the risk of a sense of betrayal when expectations of a good outcome fail. While unrealistic expectations are a hazard of a generalised trust placed in the healthcare professions, they are also a problematic feature of the public's unrealistic expectations of healthcare technology. Increasingly prevalent in advanced Western societies is a denial of personal risk in healthcare encounters and/or that a 'cure' should always be possible based on the knowledge that so many resources have been invested in technology and the constant public reminders of medical breakthroughs and advances.

Mistrust in medicine

Trust in most dimensions of healthcare is undeniably crucial but often problematic in its theoretical unpacking. Those who most conspicuously represent healthcare are the frontline clinical staff, doctors, and nurses, who in the public's imagination often symbolise the zenith of human virtue – kindness, love, compassion, and patience. With some exceptions, they are a benign presence in Western cultural narratives, so much so that even if we met them for the first time, we feel we know them fully. Akin to family members, hospital staff are almost universally regarded by the public with high, possibly idealised, and misplaced levels of trust. Why we continue to place high levels of trust in our healthcare system, or at least in medical professionals, is puzzling at times. There have been major breaches of trust across national systems ranging from individual incompetence to systemic failures of neglect, to mistreatment, mass murder, and institutional cover-ups. In the United Kingdom, the most recent and publicly disturbing of such cases relates to a former neonatal *nurse* who was convicted for the murder of seven infants and the attempted murder of six others. It is perhaps difficult to conceive of a professional role that might be invested with more trust by the public, and particularly, the parents of newborn children. Additionally alarming, when a 'whistle-blower' (a consultant paediatrician) raised concerns about the perpetrator's behaviour and the unexpected rates of infant mortality, the hospital authorities not only refused to investigate but rather, insisted that the doctor apologise to the perpetrator. We cannot know the motivations of either the killer, or the hospital administration, but we can assume that the latter was motivated to 'protect' the interests of the institution, and vicariously, their own jobs. Such cases highlight the problem in the diffusion and designation of trust. Patients may have a generalised trust about the institution of medicine and vicariously, trust its professionals. Alternatively, the trust relationship sits more directly with the individual professional at an interpersonal level but who has little control over managing trust across widespread, loosely connected actors and elements of the system. Most people remain 'loyal' to mainstream medicine, continuing to trust doctors and hospital care. Others who choose not to, preferring 'alternative' treatments may not be declaring a mistrust of mainstream medicine but rather exhibit health behaviour that is consonant with their beliefs. Western societies are progressively characterised by cultural pluralism and a fluidity of information and alternative sources of health provision. Despite mainstream demands for evidence-based treatments, many healing modalities remain relatively evidence-free and are unregulated. Others may very well exhibit distrust through deliberate avoidance. In this chapter, I will explore some of the factors that drive trust and mistrust in healthcare systems and why treatment alternatives are sought by some population sectors, and the relationship between trust, choice, and inequality.

Pluralism and choice in healthcare

The problem of delimiting the medical remains problematic (Fabrega Jr, 2020). Differences in diagnosis and treatment remain despite the movement towards evidence-based medicine in the promotion of clinical guidelines in decision-making which, theoretically at least, should lessen between and within country variations in treatment and outcomes (von dem Knesebeck et al., 2008). While societies always differ in how they understand and treat illness, they often share or borrow ideas, their health systems, organisation, and payment for health is often determined by historical circumstances and political ideologies – for example, the welfare systems of the United Kingdom and other European countries fund the healthcare of their citizens through a system of universal national insurance, which in theory at least, allows for free medical care and treatment at the point of access. Other health systems provide varying levels of free health treatment for those who cannot afford it. In all systems, many groups and individuals fall through the safety net and fail to get the care they need. In many low- and middle-income countries, the provision of healthcare is often absent completely, or precarious to say the least. Where clinical staff and facilities are non-existent or unaffordable to local people, recourse to any kind of healing, regardless of the available evidence base, fills the vacuum. In resource-depleted communities, desperation isn't a matter of trust in a particular healing modality; there are no choices to be made, individuals take whatever is on

offer. In situations of extreme patient vulnerability in which there are no alternatives of care, the patient's attitude or belief towards the physician is unlikely to be
one of 'trust'.

Resources in the form of social, educational, and financial capital offer choices.
One can choose between public and private healthcare, consult a faith-healer or
guru, or all of these. Global markets, internet advertising, and cheap flight travel
have spawned a tourist health industry, providing anything from shiny new teeth to
heart surgery, and dementia care. Although Western healthcare systems are typically
represented by an individual's relationship with a family doctor, and if warranted,
a hospital, health systems can be conceptualised as the totality of actors, beliefs,
knowledge, businesses, services, and interventions that are directed towards health
promotion, disease prevention or treatment (Kleinman, 1978). This inclusiveness
may at first seem puzzling but can be explained on several key levels. Thus, modern healthcare systems rely on transactions with multiple suppliers of goods and
services, from the very distant provider of personal protective equipment and the
pharmaceutical companies which develop new compounds to the pharmacists who
dispense them. We may also include such diverse and patient-remote professionals
as epidemiologists, health policymakers, and hospital architects. Health services
are also increasingly provided in a range of non-clinical settings such as school-
based healthcare or counselling services provided in universities and businesses.
Additionally, some health services and goods are contracted privately by the individual without mediation from a third party. These may be regulated or unregulated, increasingly obtained through a global marketplace via the internet.

Most of the healthcare is provided by informal carers in the community – family and friends. Within Kleinman's model of health systems, the latter forms the
popular sector. The *folk* sector he describes as comprising non-professional healing specialists, which may be either sacred (as performed by religious leaders)
or secular (within which sits a plethora of alternative and complementary healing
modalities such as reiki, reflexology, osteopathy). The professional sector is the
professionalised 'scientific' arena. In non-Western settings may be professionalised indigenous healing systems such as acupuncture in traditional Chinese medicine (TCM). However, increasing ethnic diversity in Western countries has paved
the way for a growth in 'indigenous' and 'alternative' professional healers and a
greater readiness of Western health consumers to obtain help from these providers.

There is evidence too that despite the advances for Western scientific medicines,
the use of complementary and alternative medicines (CAM) have increased worldwide over several decades, a popularity that shows no sign of waning (Møller et al.,
2024). However, CAM is used by many people in addition to conventional medicine rather than as a substitute and may pragmatically explore what seems to be
most effective (Barnes et al., 2004).

While modern healthcare systems tend to dominate provision, and despite
relatively high public endorsement, belief and trust in modern medicine is not
a universal given. Trust can be measured by behaviour, by the healthcare decisions that individuals make. But healthcare decisions made by individuals may

also include a recognition, or not, that they have a health problem, what kind of illness it might be, how serious it is, who and when to contact, and what kind of treatment is required. Heterogeneous health beliefs and practices are evident in increasingly multicultural societies through the provision of diverse healing alternatives; a massive alternative industry from self-help guides for almost every health and emotional problem to spiritual practitioners, and all the CAM and therapies that lie in-between. Thus, for example, one can obtain acupuncture from TCM practitioners or reiki and reflexology. Although Chinese public health services combine TCM with Western medical treatments, Western systems are unlikely to have such levels of equipoise. In the United Kingdom, the National Institute for Health and Care Excellence determined that there was insufficient, or no evidence for most CAM and would not meet these costs in the National Health Service (NHS). Where previously, treatments such as homeopathy were tolerated in NHS clinics, they quickly disappeared. However, despite the official shunning of CAM, they are still popular and in high demand, in part because of the heterogeneity in beliefs but also because of mistrust and rejection of pharmaceutical companies and the perceived unscrupulous penetration of healthcare, the heavy marketing of unproven drugs, the exaggerated claims of efficacy for many medicines which then prove to be harmful for some or all patients over time, and the readiness of physicians to prescribe harmful medication for material gains.

Pluralist health systems providing a market for different ontologies, explanatory models of illness, experiences of healthcare and preference may also increase the perceived risk in terms of choices that individuals make between alternatives within health systems. The concept of trust is only meaningful in the context of choice, but it also has salience when we acknowledge that trust is rarely compartmentalised but has dynamic and systemic aspects. While there is often a detectable ethnocentric bias in defining 'the medical' as encompassing the problems of disease and injury in a society and thus separated from legal or religious spheres and activities which, in many societies, are highly implicated in policy, diagnosis, and treatment. In many Western societies too, religion and law can influence and determine what the appropriate areas for medical attention are and/ or in what circumstances make clinical intervention possible. Thus, the extent of women's reproductive rights is often circumscribed by state legislation. So too is the legal and medical status of homosexuality and gender identity dysphoria, for example. The frameworks upon which these areas are often defined tend to arise from moral, political, or religious considerations rather than biomedical or psychiatric concerns. Moreover, socio-cultural changes emerging from the technological revolution are believed by many commentators to be responsible for the increasing prevalence of psychiatric disorders in the young; consequently, many countries seek policy and legislative responses to curb material considered harmful. Undoubtedly the internet and social media influence social attitudes and behaviours, and are harmful, but policy attention driven by social alarm provides very few solutions.

Medical conspiracy

The COVID-19 pandemic accelerated an already percolating public anxiety about an unholy alliance between state actors, healthcare industry, and the pharmaceutical companies 'big pharma'. As noted previously, trust is fragile. In 1998, an English physician and his colleagues published a somewhat methodologically flimsy case series study in the internationally prestigious medical journal *The Lancet* (Godlee et al., 2011), which suggested that the vaccine for measles, mumps, and rubella (MMR) was potentially harmful to children, predisposing them to developmental problems such as autism. Apart from the small sample that the findings were based on, there were several other critically damaging issues related to the publication, including a misrepresentation of the data, the failure to obtain ethical approval and the fact that Wakefield had failed to disclose that he was funded by lawyers hired by parents involved in lawsuits against vaccine producers. In all aspects it stank. Despite later retraction by *The Lancet* and Wakefield and colleagues disbarred from practicing medicine, the damage was done, MMR vaccination rates dropped and continue to do so, with an alarming rise in measles. Alarmingly too, is public anxiety about vaccines and the motivation of the state in promoting them, has been hijacked by 'bad actors' as a means of driving social division and resentment. In the United States an estimated 40 million people tested positive for the virus with mortality of 700,000. The enormous health and social impacts of the pandemic continue to be felt throughout every sector of society. Although the COVID-19 vaccines proved to be safe and effective if universally accepted, only 61.6% of eligible persons in the population took up the vaccine (Albrecht, 2022). A consistent body of research revealed powerful associations between conservative political and religious views and vaccination uptake in the United States and elsewhere. Albrecht (2022) noted the role of Christian nationalism, with strong ties to the Republican Party, in responding with scepticism to the COVID-19 pandemic, and the propagation of conspiracy theories. Consequently, regions with a high proportion of Trump voters had higher COVID-19-related morbidity and mortality rates than counties with fewer Trump voters.

Ethnicity and mistrust

If professional bodies, including medicine, are viewed with suspicion by minority ethnic populations, the sources of this are not difficult to detect. At times, this suspicion is bound up with unethical behaviour, corrupt practices, and misuse of power. Despite the laudable injunction embedded within the Hippocratic oath 'to do no harm', the medical profession assisted the Nazi regime in their eugenics programme and undertook barbaric experiments on adults and children. It shouldn't be forgotten either that the Nazis took inspiration from United States' policy on eugenics and popular ideas around social engineering through genetic cleansing, particularly for poor citizens in the Black community. For example, the Tuskegee Experiment led by the US Public Health Service and the Centre for Disease Control, deceived almost 400 poor African American men with syphilis, into participating in a study which left their illness untreated. Undertaken over four decades (1932–1972), the reverberations of this deceit by established medical institutions is thought to be actively felt in the rejection of COVID 19 by a large proportion of African Americans (and other minority ethnic groups). Unfortunately, there are healthcare conspiracy theories, and these are not generated through false reporting in reputable scientific journals but emerge from and disseminated by wicked social and political forces, and which are then seeded into various communities receptive to a plausibility that resonates with current anxieties and past injustices. Thus, some of the theories that have gained currency over many years hold that HIV/AIDS is a weapon of racial warfare, and that the US government encourages substance abuse among Black Americans as a means of controlling them by pushing them into poverty and prisons. Evidence indicates that a large proportion of Black Americans believe that these theories are true. Consonant with these beliefs, Black Americans are much more likely than Whites to believe that their physician will expose them to unnecessary risks, prescribe unproven medications, and provide sub-optimal care. For such reasons, Black Americans are may be relatively disinclined to trust their physicians and participate in clinical trials (Corbie-Smith et al., 2002). These findings have important implications for healthcare and good outcomes for patients. Thus, a study of attitudes and behaviours of people with HIV found that trust in care providers was associated with better engaged with services, fewer emergency room visits, increased use of antiretroviral medications, and improved reported physical and mental health. Confirming findings from community-based studies of conspiracy beliefs, more than one quarter of the study participants believed that the AIDS was a government-backed programme to kill minorities, and more than half believed that valuable AIDS information is supressed (Corbie-Smith et al., 2002).

In a study of 'medical conspiracism' using a nationally representative sample of 1351 adults, 37% of participants agreed that the Food and Drug Administration was deliberately withholding natural cures for cancer due to pharmaceutical pressure. A fifth believed that 'corporations' censored public health information about data linking cell phones to cancer or that physicians still pursued the vaccination of children despite knowing such vaccines to be dangerous (Oliver & Wood, 2014). Participants classified as 'High conspiracists' were individuals more likely to buy organic foods and use herbal supplements and less likely to use protective care or have annual check-ups. Controlling for socioeconomic status, paranoia, and general social estrangement the authors found that medical conspiracism remained a strong predictor of these health behaviours.

For most of human history, humans lived as hunter-gatherers in small tribal groups, alert to the threat from animal predators and competition not just from other groups but the danger posed by the formation of coalitions within one's one group. The need to anticipate competition by others for scarce resources and be alert to internal and external dangers, suggests that a pervasive sense of trust might pose an existential threat. Quite the opposite, a degree of paranoia might just provide the individual with a competitive edge for survival. Too much paranoia however, and the individual might have problems in forming relationships and alliances, not a great reproductive position and hence, not a good evolutionary strategy at the extreme end of paranoia, borne out by evidence that suggests that individuals with paranoid traits have lower reproductive success (Raihani & Bell, 2019). In the realm of a psychiatric disorder, severity or actual pathology is determined by the individual's ability to continue functioning – to work and maintain relationships, for example. In addition to schizophrenia, bipolar disorder, and major depressive disorders,

Paranoia and conspiracy theories

Healthcare systems are vulnerable to mistrust by some sections of the public because they are regarded suspiciously as instruments of power, a belief increasingly translated into socio-political anxieties about control over lives and bodies. There is a strong evolutionary case to be made for the benefits of paranoia, commonly regarded as a symptom of severe mental illness but which can encompass phenomena such as a mild feeling that other people may be seeking to cause one harm, through to quite delusional ideas that there are dark forces in conspiracy against you. The literature offers a range of dimensions none of which Freeman (2007) a leading authority on delusional ideation, suggests are necessary or sufficient, but with cumulative endorsement provides more likelihood of a delusion being present. Thus, whether the belief is implausible, groundless, intensely held, unshared by others, distressing and preoccupying are strongly indicative of a delusion. Key in any discussion of delusion is that there is considerable individual variability in the features of delusional experience and demonstrate complex, multi-dimensional experiences.

Thus, the variety is in the content of persecutory thoughts, such as the type and timing of threat, the focus of the harm, the motivation of the persecutor. In defining persecutory ideation, 'the individual believes that harm is occurring, or is going to occur, to him or her, and that the persecutor has the intention to cause harm' and these should be distinguished from commonly held anxious thoughts (Freeman & Garety, 2000).

Trust in healthcare agencies and professionals is complex and uncertain. For example, with the complicity of many thousands of family doctors and an extraordinary marketing campaign, opioid prescriptions in the United States rocketed, resulting in a fourfold increase from 1990 to 2010. This was partly due to an overly trusting acceptance of physician (and pharmacist) integrity and inadequate regulation of their industries within a few years, North America witnessed an unprecedented use of highly potent opioids for conditions that would normally have been considered inappropriate. While thousands of deaths occurred through opioid overdosing, millions more became addicted or harmed vicariously. Thus, the cost of family breakdown, crime, unemployment, and violent behaviour through inappropriate opioid prescribing by health professionals is vast, possibly incalculable. It is estimated that in excess of 300,000 Americans have died from overdoses of prescription opioids since 2000 (Humphreys et al., 2022; Patel et al., 2018). While serial killers have emerged within general medicine, to my knowledge no psychiatrist has.

Until the emergence of Enlightenment rationalism, medicine as widely practiced in Western societies was rooted in religious organisations and generally, little more than a branch of metaphysics underpinned by guesswork, poisoning, and butchery. However, outside of the development of Western systems of medicine, the development of healing practices is universal (Fabrega Jr, 2020). This being so, different societies and cultural groups construct healing resources and institutions from the materials available to them, and the environments from which the sickness and potential for healing arises. Heart disease, type 2 diabetes, and cancer may not be very prevalent in sub-Saharan Africa but remain major health problems in modern Western economies, largely created by the food industry and for which a vast array of scientific medical and psychological energies, research, and intervention has been assembled to combat or manage such diseases, with little impact.

Medicalisation of human distress

Western technological societies appear to have created an expectation among their populations that material and scientific solutions exist for all problems, providing the availability of finances. However, there remains scepticism about claims of scientific deliverance from human need and suffering (Good & Good, 1980). Many commentators from diverse and eclectic orientations struggle against what is consider as a form of medical colonialism, an expanding intrusion of professionalism into the natural stuff of human problems (Illich, 1977).

However, it is accepted that medicine more generally, and psychiatry specifically, have long been accused of hegemonic ambitions in many spheres of the human condition, across the broad domains and events of what it is to be human – birth, emotional development, morality, sickness, and death. It has been defined by Davis (2010) as 'the process by which medical definitions and practices are applied to behaviours, psychological phenomena and somatic experiences not previously within the conceptual or therapeutic scope of medicine'. While medicalisation has existed in some form or other, for instance in the replacing of supernatural or moral explanations and treatments with those based on psychiatric concepts and pharmaceutical treatments, the concern across many sectors, views medicine as having an unchecked appetite for appropriating areas of life that belong more correctly to the personal realm. So, while in some areas of living, a medical definition and approach, was a liberation of the individual harsh and pointless judgements, in many other aspects, medicine was regarded as intruding unnecessarily into human responses to suffering. It is not just that medicine offered an alternative response, but that that it obliterated significant functions of human experience, including the benefits of suffering (Illich, 1977) and the intimacy of human contact in caring. Other critiques of establishment medicine emerged from within Marxist, feminist, anti-racist, and LGBTQ movements, and very often within psychiatry itself.

Health systems and personhood

In the medical sociology literature, the human experiences of sadness, grief, loneliness, and dying, once the domain of spirituality (Durà-Vilà et al., 2013), are viewed as encroached upon up by an expanding medical hegemony.[3] In some respects, the concerns about the motivations and direction of travel for healthcare appear to have some basis. Certainly, the conglomeration or network of relationships termed by Barbara Ehrenreich as the 'medical-industrial complex' with its considerable expansion across sectors new sectors of 'need', vast profits, and deep political influence, provokes anxieties now just related to conflicts of interest but that the medical industry may not be operating in the best interests of the patient. There is insufficient space to deal with this issue adequately here, but while acknowledging that the development of new pharmaceutical compounds and technology is hugely risky and expensive, the pharmaceutical and healthcare industries, even within the United Kingdom's NHS, increasingly derive profits that simply do not accord with usual theories of markets.

As far back as 1980, Relman (1980) writing in the *New England Journal of Medicine*, described the absurdities in the US healthcare system. Because healthcare technology requires a level of investment that is generally beyond the reach of most non-profit organisations, private entrepreneurs have stepped in to fill this gap in 'services efficiently and an acceptable level of quality'. What would normally be expected in free markets is that the disciplining forces of competition and consumer choice would drive private entrepreneurs to offer better and varied products and services for less than could be provided by non-profit organisations or by government-run services. Thus, large for-profit organisations are incentivised to control costs through better management and can benefit from economies of scale. Of course, this couldn't emerge in healthcare, simply because health doesn't operate just as other goods and services do. People desire the best healthcare available and will pay whatever they can to obtain it. Moreover, most people in the United States obtain their healthcare through insurance companies and aren't consumers as it is usually conceptualised – in other words, another agency at some level of distance and abstraction is seeking services on their behalf. In addition, the decision-making of patients unlike other consumers is largely directed by the information provided by doctors – they do not actively choose their healthcare plans and treatment.

The conundrum that Relman posed 40 years ago persists – that while healthcare costs much more in the United States, the outcomes for people across the lifespan are much worse than elsewhere (Emanuel, 2018; Starfield, 2000). While the NHS in the United Kingdom appears to achieve better outcomes for less expenditure, it increasingly opens its system to private healthcare providers and entrepreneurs which tend to 'skim' the most lucrative services while leaving the 'money-draining' chronic care to the public provider. The same is true about high-risk but much needed pharmaceuticals for people with relatively rare conditions. The market does not meet these needs because there is no financial incentive to do so. Additionally, the private system employs clinicians who have been trained through public funding, and thus are able to gain higher profits. Another issue raised by Relman, and an increasingly prescient one, is the increasing reliance of healthcare providers on specific procedures and technology while excluding personal care. This is a problem no longer peculiar to private healthcare.

Disconnection and technology

Healing is as much art as science. The emergence and maintenance of patient–doctor trust is predicated on the patients' confidence that the clinician possesses the appropriate training and skills, they have competencies related to the desired outcome. Mostly, the patient cannot be sure that these competencies are in place, they trust the healthcare employers have done due diligence in appointing skilled and qualified people. However, patient trust is most obviously generated by the emotional, empathic qualities that the clinician is able to portray authentically and convincingly. However, in various studies on the core components of quality care, clinicians tend to promote technical skills above intrinsic qualities, the reverse of patients and families (Flocke et al., 2002). Compassion, considered a major determinant of patient satisfaction and related to quality in healthcare incorporates virtues and their expression in honesty, kindness, helpfulness, non-judgmental attitudes, and behaviours such as smile, touch, care, support, and flexibility (Singh et al., 2018). Although most of these qualities have a universal appeal and are important elements in therapeutic engagement, a clinician's 'lack of time' is consistently reported as the main barrier to compassionate care. Distilling this further, increasing healthcare costs and scarcity of human resources place restrictions on the provision of compassionate, person-centred care. It has become a luxury not an essential.

The use of digital technology, including AI diagnostics, biological sensor monitoring, assisted surgery, and robotics, to name a few, is well advanced in diverse healthcare systems, and governments and industry are optimistically aligned in the potential of AI's to deliver precision and efficiency in healthcare, even though this vision may not be in tune with various commentators and the public.[4] The resource-intense nature of personal care makes healthcare technology an attractive investment by government, and of course, industry. Thus, there is a tendency to think that advanced technology will assist in the early detection and management of illnesses. Throughout the 20th century, natural human processes and events from birth to death have been transferred from domestic to institutional settings where medical intervention is pushed to its logical end, leading to fragmentation of care and loss of personhood. Patient isolation through care regimentation is now commonplace in acute and skilled nursing care facilities. As one commentator puts it, 'Care for the dying person, "system by system, organ by organ", as is typical in institutional settings, fragments the dying process into a series of medical events' (O'Connell, 1996).[5] The attendant motivations and risks involved medical intervention in natural processes once again provoke questions about inherent ambiguities in healthcare outcomes and just who the intended beneficiaries might be.

Where in the process does patient trust reside? Quite possibly it is an irrelevance within the abstract logic of systematised rather than personalised care.

In critical care situations, where once humans sat in vigil with a relative or friend, acclimatising and comforting, clinicians now glance dispassionately at a monitor bleeping vital signal, as if that is what matters. In the interests of efficiency, professionals lack the necessary time and skills to address spiritual and existential issues of importance to the patient. These may require good communication skills and a flexibility of time that are not aligned with current hospital routines (Murray et al., 2004). As Pilgrim and colleagues (2011, p. 113) noted, the introduction of managerial practices eliminates the satisfactory building of interpersonal trust between the patient and the hospital. Central to this relationship is the desire of the patient 'to be seen', to be cared for rather, than a passive body, the vital signs of which are monitored through a machine, regardless of its sophistication.

Notes

1 However, our findings suggest that people with severe mental illness have a more rapid onset due to multiple risk factors. The presence of more symptoms may allow for a heightened awareness and earlier detection than general hospital patients.
2 This is as much true in traditional healing as in Western medical systems (Zuma et al., 2016).
3 Ivan Illich argues that dying and suffering are meaningful aspects of life upon which humans must contemplate and accept. Medicalisation, insists on a suspension of the inevitable, encouraging an expectation of intervention. Humans are pushed further from acceptance. Depression too may be an aspect of the human condition that perhaps could and should be tolerated and out of which may come understanding and change. Psychiatric pharmacological intervention creates or at least in part, is founded in the belief that we all have the right to happiness.
4 At the time of writing, Western governments and industry have been responding to concerns from experts and public about the dangers of AI, some of which relate to the inherent dangers of super-intelligent systems developing autonomy, making decisions that are outside the control of human agents, and which be endangering to life. Less dramatically science fiction perhaps, but nevertheless threatening, is the threat of bad agents hacking healthcare systems for monetary gain or as a weapon in warfare.
5 Moreover, institutionalised care may diminish the compassion of clinical staff who come to view the dying person more as an object of academic interest than as a human whose spiritual needs may transcend physical ones. Thus, existential and spiritual issues have become marginalised in the palliative and supportive care of cancer patients. However, as concepts of adequate supportive care move beyond a focus on pain and physical symptom control, existential and spiritual issues such as meaning, hope, and spirituality in general are gradually receiving attention from supportive care clinicians and clinical researchers.

References

Albrecht, D. (2022). Vaccination, politics and COVID-19 impacts. *BMC Public Health*, *22*(1), 96. https://doi.org/10.1186/s12889-021-12432-x
Albrecht, D. E. (2022). COVID-19 in rural America: Impacts of politics and disadvantage. *Rural Sociology*, *87*(1), 94–118.

Attar, R., Berg Johansen, M., Valentin, J. B., Aagaard, J., & Jensen, S. E. (2017). Treatment following myocardial infarction in patients with schizophrenia. *PLOS One, 12*(12), e0189289. https://doi.org/10.1371/journal.pone.0189289

Barbalet, J. (2009). A characterization of trust, and its consequences. *Theory and Society, 38*(4), 367–382. http://www.jstor.org/stable/40345659

Barnes, P. M., Powell-Griner, E., McFann, K., & Nahin, R. L. (2004). Complementary and alternative medicine use among adults: United States, 2002. *Advance Data,* (343), 1–19.

Benedetti, F., Maggi, G., Lopiano, L., Lanotte, M., Rainero, I., Vighetti, S., & Pollo, A. (2003). Open versus hidden medical treatments: The patient's knowledge about a therapy affects the therapy outcome. *Prevention & Treatment, 6*(1), 1a.

Cabana, M. D., & Jee, S. H. (2004). Does continuity of care improve patient outcomes? *Journal of Family Practice, 53*(12), 974–980.

Colagiuri, B., Schenk, L. A., Kessler, M. D., Dorsey, S. G., & Colloca, L. (2015). The placebo effect: From concepts to genes. *Neuroscience, 307,* 171–190. https://doi.org/10.1016/j.neuroscience.2015.08.017

Cook, K. S., Kramer, R. M., Thom, D. H., Stepanikova, I., Mollborn, S. B., & Cooper, R. M. (2004). Trust and distrust in patient-physician relationships: Perceived determinants of high- and low-trust relationships in managed care settings. In M. Kramer & K. Cook (Eds.), *Trust and distrust in organizations: Dilemmas and approaches*. Russell Sage.

Corbie-Smith, G., Thomas, S. B., & St George, D. M. (2002). Distrust, race, and research. *Archives of Internal Medicine, 162*(21), 2458–2463. https://doi.org/10.1001/archinte.162.21.2458

Davis, J. E. (2010). Medicalization, social control, and the relief of suffering. In W. C. Cockerham (Ed.), *The Blackwell companion to medical sociology* (pp. 211–241). Wiley.

Durà-Vilà, G., Littlewood, R., & Leavey, G. (2013). Depression and the medicalization of sadness: Conceptualization and recommended help-seeking. *International Journal of Social Psychiatry, 59*(2), 165–175. https://doi.org/10.1177/0020764011430037

Emanuel, E. J. (2018). The real cost of the US health care system. *JAMA, 319*(10), 983–985. https://doi.org/10.1001/jama.2018.1151

Fabrega Jr, H. (2020). Evolution of sickness and healing. In *Evolution of sickness and healing*. University of California Press.

Fabrega, H. J. (1997). *Evolution of sickness and healing*. University of California Press.

Flocke, S. A., Miller, W. L., & Crabtree, B. F. (2002). Relationships between physician practice style, patient satisfaction, and attributes of primary care. *Journal of Family Practice, 51*(10), 835–840.

Freeman, D. (2007). Suspicious minds: The psychology of persecutory delusions. *Clinical Psychology Review, 27*(4), 425–457. https://doi.org/10.1016/j.cpr.2006.10.004

Freeman, D., & Garety, P. A. (2000). Comments on the content of persecutory delusions: Does the definition need clarification? *British Journal of Clinical Psychology, 39*(4), 407–414.

Friedson, E. (1960). Client control and medical practice. *American Journal of Sociology, 65,* 374–382.

Giddens, A. (1991). *Modernity and self-identity: Self and society in the late modern age*. Polity Press.

Godlee, F., Smith, J., & Marcovitch, H. (2011). Wakefield's article linking MMR vaccine and autism was fraudulent: Clear evidence of falsification of data should now close the door on this damaging vaccine scare. *BMJ: British Medical Journal, 342*(7788), 64–66. http://www.jstor.org/stable/25766651

Good, B. J., & Good, M. J. D. (1980). The meaning of symptoms: A cultural hermeneutic model for clinical practice. In L. Eisenberg & A. Kleinman (Ed.), *The relevance of social science for medicine* (pp. 165–196). Springer.

Green, J., & Goldwyn, R. (2002). Annotation: Attachment disorganisation and psychopathology: New findings in Attachment research and their potential implications for developmental psychopathology in childhood. *Journal of Child Psychology and Psychiatry*, *43*(7), 835–846. https://doi.org/10.1111/1469-7610.00102

Hall, M. A., Dugan, E., Zheng, B., & Mishra, A. K. (2001). Trust in physicians and medical institutions: What is it, can it be measured, and does it matter? *Milbank Quarterly*, *79*(4), 613–639. https://doi.org/10.1111/1468-0009.00223

Hart, W., Albarracín, D., Eagly, A. H., Brechan, I., Lindberg, M. J., & Merrill, L. (2009). Feeling validated versus being correct: A meta-analysis of selective exposure to information. *Psychological Bulletin*, *135*(4), 555–588. https://doi.org/10.1037/a0015701

Humphreys, K., Shover, C. L., Andrews, C. M., Bohnert, A. S., Brandeau, M. L., Caulkins, J. P., Chen, J. H., Cuéllar, M.-F., Hurd, Y. L., & Juurlink, D. N. (2022). Responding to the opioid crisis in North America and beyond: Recommendations of the Stanford–Lancet Commission. *The Lancet*, *399*(10324), 555–604.

Illich, I. (1977). *Limits to medicine: Medical nemesis, the expropriation of health*. Harmondsworth.

Kaptchuk, T. J., Friedlander, E., Kelley, J. M., Sanchez, M. N., Kokkotou, E., Singer, J. P., Kowalczykowski, M., Miller, F. G., Kirsch, I., & Lembo, A. J. (2010). Placebos without deception: A randomized controlled trial in irritable bowel syndrome. *PLOS One*, *5*(12), e15591.

Kleinman, A. (1978). Concepts and a model for the comparison of medical systems as cultural systems. *Social Science & Medicine. Part B: Medical Anthropology*, *12*, 85–93. https://doi.org/10.1016/0160-7987(78)90014-5

Luhmann, N. (1988). Familiarity, confidence, trust: Problems and alternatives. In D. Gambetta (Ed.), *Trust: Making and breaking cooperative relations* (pp. 94–107). University of Oxford.

McCarter, R., Rosato, M., Thampi, A., Barr, R., & Leavey, G. (2023). Physical health disparities and severe mental illness: A longitudinal comparative cohort study using hospital data in Northern Ireland. *European Psychiatry*, 2023;*66*(1):e70. doi:10.1192/j.eurpsy.2023.2441.

Mechanic, D. (1998). Public trust and initiatives for new health care partnerships. *Milbank Quarterly*, *76*(2), 281–302. https://doi.org/10.1111/1468-0009.00089

Møller, S. R., Ekholm, O., & Christensen, A. I. (2024). Trends in the use of complementary and alternative medicine between 1987 and 2021 in Denmark. *BMC Complementary Medicine and Therapies*, *24*(1), 23. https://doi.org/10.1186/s12906-023-04327-8

Murray, S. A., Kendall, M., Boyd, K., Worth, A., & Benton, T. F. (2004). Exploring the spiritual needs of people dying of lung cancer or heart failure: A prospective qualitative interview study of patients and their carers. *Palliative Medicine*, *18*(1), 39–45.

O'Connell, L. J. (1996). Changing the culture of dying. A new awakening of spirituality in America heightens sensitivity to needs of dying persons. *Health Programme*, *77*(6), 16–20.

Oliver, J. E., & Wood, T. (2014). Medical conspiracy theories and health behaviors in the United States. *JAMA Internal Medicine*, *174*(5), 817–818. https://doi.org/10.1001/jamainternmed.2014.190

Patel, V., Saxena, S., Lund, C., Thornicroft, G., Baingana, F., Bolton, P., Chisholm, D., Collins, P. Y., Cooper, J. L., Eaton, J., Herrman, H., Herzallah, M. M., Huang, Y., Jordans, M. J. D., Kleinman, A., Medina-Mora, M. E., Morgan, E., Niaz, U., Omigbodun, O., ... & UnÜtzer, J. (2018). The Lancet Commission on global mental health and sustainable development. *Lancet*, *392*(10157), 1553–1598. https://doi.org/10.1016/s0140-6736(18)31612-x

Pearson, S. D., & Raeke, L. H. (2000). Patients' trust in physicians: Many theories, few measures, and little data. *Journal of General Internal Medicine* *15*(7), 509–513. https://doi.org/10.1046/j.1525-1497.2000.11002.x

Pilgrim, D., Tomasini, F., & Yassilev, I. (2011). *Examining trust in health care: A multidisciplinary perspective.* Palgrave Macmillan.

Porter, R. (1997). *The greatest benefit to mankind: A medical history of humanity from antiquity to the present.* Fontana Press.

Raihani, N. J., & Bell, V. (2019). An evolutionary perspective on paranoia. *Nature Human Behaviour, 3*(2), 114–121. https://doi.org/10.1038/s41562-018-0495-0

Relman, A. S. (1980). The new medical-industrial complex. *New England Journal of Medicine, 303*(17), 963–970. https://doi.org/10.1056/nejm198010233031703

Rhodes, R., & Strain, J. J. (2000). Trust and transforming medical institutions. *Cambridge Quarterly of Healthcare Ethics, 9*(2), 205–217. https://doi.org/10.1017/s096318010090207x

Rydgren, J. (2012). Beliefs. In P. Hedström & P. Bearman (Eds.), *The Oxford handbook of analytical sociology* (pp. 72–93). Oxford University Press.

Scheunemann, L. P., & White, D. B. (2011). The ethics and reality of rationing in medicine. *Chest, 140*(6), 1625–1632. https://doi.org/10.1378/chest.11-0622

Schoen, C., Osborn, R., Huynh, P. T., Doty, M., Davis, K., Zapert, K., & Peugh, J. (2004). Primary care and health system performance: Adults' experiences in five countries. *Health Aff (Millwood), Suppl Web Exclusives,* W4-487–503. https://doi.org/10.1377/hlthaff.w4.487

Singh, P., King-Shier, K., & Sinclair, S. (2018). The colours and contours of compassion: A systematic review of the perspectives of compassion among ethnically diverse patients and healthcare providers. *PLOS One, 13*(5), e0197261. https://doi.org/10.1371/journal.pone.0197261

Skinner, B., Leavey, G., & Rothi, D. (2021). Managerialism and teacher professional identity: Impact on well-being among teachers in the UK. *Educational Review, 73*(1), 1–16. https://doi.org/10.1080/00131911.2018.1556205

Starfield, B. (2000). Is US health really the best in the world? *JAMA, 284*(4), 483–485. https://doi.org/10.1001/jama.284.4.483

Strech, D., Persad, G., Marckmann, G., & Danis, M. (2009). Are physicians willing to ration health care? Conflicting findings in a systematic review of survey research. *Health Policy, 90*(2-3), 113–124. https://doi.org/10.1016/j.healthpol.2008.10.013

von dem Knesebeck, O., Bönte, M., Siegrist, J., Marceau, L., Link, C., Arber, S., Adams, A., & McKinlay, J. (2008). Country differences in the diagnosis and management of coronary heart disease – A comparison between the US, the UK and Germany. *BMC Health Services Research, 8*(1), 198. https://doi.org/10.1186/1472-6963-8-198

Zuma, T., Wight, D., Rochat, T., & Moshabela, M. (2016). The role of traditional health practitioners in rural KwaZulu-Natal, South Africa: Generic or mode specific? *BMC Complementary and Alternative Medicine, 16*(1), 304. https://doi.org/10.1186/s12906-016-1293-8

Chapter 7

Mistrust in Psychiatry

Criticism of psychiatry and psychiatrists has been a consistent feature of cultural discourse over the past century. Often a source of public fear, disguised as mockery and amusement, the institution is regularly obliged to defend its professional knowledge, integrity, and processes unlike any other medical professions. The disrespect and mistrust it attracts as a discipline does not align with its task, in terms of the prevalence of mental illness and the associated costs to the individual and society. Thus, the economic consequences of mental disorders are considerable through the direct medical costs of care and treatment, outpatient visits, and hospitalisation. There are major indirect costs too, through unemployment and welfare benefits, reduced educational attainment and low productivity due to disability and absenteeism. A recent study indicated that the global economic value associated with this burden is estimated at about USD 5 trillion (Patel et al., 2016). Given the importance of psychiatry's task, it is hard to understand the relative disrespect (stigma) for the profession in public and cultural discourses. Some of the explanation can be found in its history. A relatively recent branch of medicine, it has long struggled to shake off its colourful, often abhorrent, foundations. Discarding its wilder beliefs and practices, it began to assert its legitimacy in the 20th century but is still regularly mired by internal disputes about the aetiology, treatment, and potential cures for mental illnesses. The discipline divides on whether the origins of disorders such as depression or schizophrenia are to be located in the brain or the mind, in the environment and society, or in our genes and biology. Its knowledge claims and scientific basis may therefore be undermined within its own professional sphere. However, it is sometimes forgotten that the now-respectable branches of medicine that primarily deal with physical disorders, cannot be viewed with nostalgic fondness at their benign naivety. Medicine's historical pathway to respectability too is strewn with what might be considered by contemporary values and understanding, as criminality, butchery, and dishonesty of every sort. Even today, highly professionalised, and regulated institutions make alarming mistakes, and malevolent clinicians are brought within the criminal justice system for sadistic and murderous acts.

The roots of psychiatry as a discipline are not obviously 'medical', but then again, medicine's past was not recognisably medical either. Religious beliefs and

DOI: 10.4324/9781003326687-7

institutions played a major role in both. However, the separate quest for trust in psychiatry has always been vexed by questions of scientific legitimacy, and binary internal disciplinary conflicts between 'mind' and 'brain'-biological versus social determinants of mental illness. Whereas general medicine is underpinned by huge investments by the pharmacological industry, and significant scientific and technological advances, psychiatry has few triumphs. Over the past century, the institution heralded all kinds of scientific breakthroughs in the physical or chemical reformation of the brain, most of which have proved to be ineffective at best, and brutally destructive at worst. Increasingly mental health services are dependent on pharmacological solutions to human distress while depression, self-harm, and suicide rates appear to rise defiantly. These sorts of brick walls continue to undercut confidence in the discipline.

In this chapter, I will review relatively old critiques of psychiatry, but still relevant and expanding, concerning the discipline's potential overreach and intrusion into aspects of the human condition. A significant proportion of the mistrust in psychiatry is due to a residual institutional stigma, a leftover from the days of public asylums that continue to inhabit the public imagination (Scull, 1977). The professional activities that provoke mistrust in psychiatry are concerns that it may not be acting in the best interests of all people. Specifically, that psychiatry might be containing rather than curing, or 'curing' what isn't sick. Thus, the patient's evaluation of motivation is a major aspect of interpersonal and institutional trust. This is the intersection of inequality and social discrimination and an ambivalence among sections of the community about the 'true' role of psychiatry and the discipline's cultural competencies in the diagnostic assessment and management of minoritised populations.

For others, the potential for ambivalence in the function of psychiatry is ever present as I explore through the increasingly socially visible issue of gender dysphoria and how the current cultural anxieties that suffuse the issue of gender spill over into the provision and management of services.

Psychiatry and power

Much of the criticism against psychiatry that developed in the mid-20th century was from 'survivors' of the asylum system, people who had been incarcerated against their will, and subjected to invasive procedures, including electroconvulsive treatment, leucotomy, and insulin-induced coma (Porter, 1997; Scull, 2019). The view that 'zombified' patients were preferential to distressed ones seems an extraordinary breach of medical ethics but, it would appear, commonly acceptable to psychiatry and the public at the time. That much of the armamentarium employed in psychiatric hospitals over the 20th century have been dumped, the efficacy of such interventions widely discredited, has raised questions about the alacrity with which they were accepted in the first place. Critics suggest that such interventions were accepted by a willing psychiatry because they had a scientific appearance and that they simply gave psychiatrists something to do.

Their narratives of past and current patients about coercive overreach in the psychiatric profession, aligned with the counter-cultural zeitgeist of the 1960s and 1970s; resistance to a maddening socio-political system and violent, repressive state machinery (Arendt, 1970). Much of the anti-psychiatric discourse suggested that psychiatry was simply another state tool of oppression, a 'softer' but more subtly cruel branch of policing which facilitated the incarceration of people antipathetic to the establishment. More than that, ideas, beliefs, and attitudes considered dangerous or non-conforming to societal norms could be suppressed or expunged by labelling and detaining the individuals deemed to be mad. Szasz (1973, pp. 205–206), in vehement opposition to psychiatry's pathologisation of homosexuality, writes, 'It is clear that psychiatrists have a vested interest in diagnosing as mentally ill many people as possible, just as inquisitors had in branding them as heretics. The "conscientious" psychiatrist authenticates himself as a competent medical man by holding all sexual deviants (and all kinds of other people, perhaps all of mankind, as Karl Menninger would have it) as mentally ill, just as the "conscientious" inquisitor authenticated himself as a faithful Christian by holding that homosexuals (and all kinds of other people) were heretics. We must realise that in situations of this kind we are confronted, not with scientific problems to be solved, but with social roles to be confirmed'. Szasz then goes on to say that the state gives power to the psychiatrist, in the same way that Church gave power to the inquisitor.[1]

In the same year as Szasz's book, *The Manufacture of Madness* was published, an academic publication by David Rosenham appeared in *Science*. Called *Being Sane in Insane Places* and published in *Science*, it injected yet more controversy into an already contested space about the reality of psychiatric practice, the validity of psychiatry as a medical science, and the function of asylums. Rosenham, a professor of psychology and law, tutored some of his college students to act as pseudo-patients, expressing vague symptoms, mostly hearing voices and asking existential questions about the meaning and purpose of life. Without much difficulty, apparently, the pseudo-patients duped the psychiatric staff who incarcerated them for an average of 19 days, following a diagnosis of schizophrenia. Once inside they behaved 'normally'. They were all eventually discharged, diagnosed with *schizophrenia in remission*. Much commented upon was the observation that only the 'real' patients had any inkling as to the deception. Rosenham's main criticism was not that the sham patients were wrongly detained, but that the psychiatrists had made a diagnostic 'leap' from the students' hallucinations to a diagnosis of schizophrenia. Today, the possibility of such an easy access to many weeks hospital stay would raise the eyebrows of most hospital managers. At the time, the widespread and damming conclusion among commentators was that psychiatry itself was a sham.[2]

This view of psychiatry as an adjunct to an oppressive state expressed by people like Szasz who, despite being a psychiatrist, voiced concerns about psychiatry that persist about the medicalisation of emotional and interpersonal problems, the willingness, as he saw it, for psychiatry to intrude into, and colonise, all aspects of human behaviour – pathologising individuals and groups through the authority of diagnosis. Psychiatry as a branch of medicine deals with mental suffering, symptoms brought often about by disruptions that are not easily observable or traceable to bodily disorders, even though they may have profound bodily effects. Much of the processes in the recognition, reporting, classification, and management of such disorders, as noted previously, are often contentious, particularly in relation to cultural differences in the presentation and interpretation of symptoms, but also due to accusations of general psychiatric overreach and misdiagnosis. Andrew Scull makes the link between Rosenham's academic exposé of psychiatry's inability to differentiate between the sane and the insane, and the arrival of the *Diagnostic and Statistical Manual of Mental Disorders* (*DSM 111*), skilfully shepherded in by Robert Spitzer, based, apparently, on rather flimsy data and unpublished evidence. The intention of the DSM was to develop a manual of mental disorders, each with a checklist of defined symptoms that would facilitate the universal reliability of psychiatric diagnoses. Scull argues, as others have done, that what the DSM couldn't do was increase the *validity* of these diagnoses – that they often didn't correspond with genuine diseases. 'it paid no attention whether the entities existed in nature, independent of psychiatric judgement, being satisfied with concocting labels that were consistently applied' (Scull, 2019, p. 173).

Szasz raised philosophical, moral, and legal questions about the psychiatric erosion of human agency. Importantly, while acknowledging the 'suffering' of individuals he questioned the legitimacy of psychiatric diagnoses, preferring to recognise this suffering as 'problems in living' which were not the monopolistic domain of the psychiatric profession, and moreover, could only be attended to voluntarily rather than coercion. Indeed, Szasz questioned the legitimacy of 'mental illnesses' as genuine diseases, using television to draw an analogy between the content of a television programme and its technical delivery; that is, it's impossible to improve the content of the programme by calling upon the services of the engineer. However, while the mental problems of the individual are often the consequences of social circumstances and events outside the body, regardless of the genetic components, psychiatry as we have noted, seeks to burnish its biological credentials, free of sociocultural contexts.

While many of Szasz's libertarian arguments are problematic, we can nevertheless acknowledge various important concerns about psychiatry as an overreaching institution of 'soft power', its questionable support for establishment perspectives, and the pathologising of non-normative behaviours. On this last point, it is worth remembering that homosexuality was considered a disorder within the *DSM-11* and not removed until 1986. That it continues to be 'treated' as such by so-called 'conversion therapy' within religious milieu indicates the enduring power of labelling and the co-opting of medicine in support of mistreatment (King et al., 2004). Of course, while he didn't examine ethnicity per se, Szasz's arguments resonate with the belief that psychiatry has been used as a coercive instrument, co-opted by the welfare state into dealing with the anger and resistance within the black community in the United Kingdom.

Psychiatric power and mistrust

Our understanding of the legitimising power of psychiatry is perhaps best supported through the work of, Michel Foucault, who like Szasz questioned the biological underpinnings for psychiatric disorders and the scientific assertions of the discipline, but rather, that the diagnoses developed and applied are little more than moral evaluations that serve to ameliorate anxieties of dominant classes. Foucault speaks of 'disciplinary power', distinguishing it from brute dominating power exerted through force and punishment but rather a more subtle internalisation of beliefs and values – the creation of an ideological ambience in which the truths obtain popular acceptance of 'how things are'. In this sense, power operates invisibly in the background creating its own legitimacy, its own sense of the truth. The enlightenment encouraged a rationalist worldview that seeks technocratic solutions to social challenges. It is not that all such solutions themselves are motivated by malice or even that they are inherently wrong, though many are, it is simply that they are inherently aspects of a technological culture with often unquestioned assumptions about the legitimacy of the response.

Psychology and psychiatry, through a Foucauldian history, only materialise as medical disciplines from the asylum systems in Europe and the United States, for which, the incarceration of people deemed insane, was an efficiently purgative approach to the needs of the industrial revolution. As Bracken and Thomas (2010) suggest, 'All are the products of the operation of power/knowledge. All involve authority, goals, and discipline, and are linked to the development of our modern economy and culture. In this culture, problems with our behaviours, relationships, beliefs, and sexualities show up not as religious, spiritual, or moral issues, but as technical problems that are open to examination, classification, analysis, and intervention by suitably trained experts'. A similar point is made by Charles Taylor in his concern for a 'therapeutic' turn in modern societies, shifting from a religious and moral ethos in which human behaviour must be guided and assessed by soteriological concerns – the requirements of earthly actions for salvation in the afterlife – and therefore, bound up with very Roman Catholic concepts of sin, suffering, and atonement. However, it is found in almost all religions, and noticeably expressed in Protestant traditions in the spirit of Calvinism, guided by restraint and self-denial. The therapeutic turn as described by Taylor and others arrived with the advent of capitalism, secularism, and individualism. Although some commentators have regarded this as a liberating, an opportunity for an authentic self over the tyranny of the moral demands of the community, others including Taylor observed narcissism whereby individuals, divested of commitments to the community are now as Giddens also noted focussed on self-improvement and the 'project of the self' (Giddens, 1991). What were once moral concerns are transformed into therapeutic issues. Thus, a wide spectrum of diametrically opposed problems from sexual timidity to sexual promiscuity, for example, are now 'treatable' – requiring only the individual's self-assessment of their salience to unhappiness. In Western societies, Foucault suggests that psychiatry through an increasing individualism in which the horrors and challenges experienced by citizens are now considered to be the discrete products of faulty minds rather than influenced by supernatural forces.

It is true that disciplinary power is also noticeably located in other branches of medicine, not just psychiatry. Moral evaluations of patients appear in sexual and reproductive health, and an array of public health interventions related to cardio-vascular and endocrine health – alcohol and substance misuse, diet and nutrition, and exercise. However, it is psychiatry that is most easily vulnerable to cultural uncertainty, subjective interpretation, and ideological manipulation. Hence, the long-standing and highly contested arena of the prevalence of mental illness in minority ethnic communities, especially in the relationships between black people, the diagnosis of schizophrenia, and mental health services, in which trust, and mis-trust play a major role.

Complexity and diversity

As noted previously, modern Western societies are characterised by increasingly complex diversity and pluralism in communities, beliefs, and knowledge. In whom one places trust when one becomes ill is often dependent on its appraisal and rec-ognition as an illness by self and other people in that community. The highly sub-jective and concealed nature of a mental illness and its symptoms, say depression, relative to that of a physical illness, such as diabetes, adds further complexity to the process of recognition. The symptoms of diabetes are readily traceable to a bodily location and identifying the problem and potential treatments for such symptoms are available. Fellow sufferers tend not to be shy in offering personal experience and various orthodox and unorthodox interventions. If symptoms persist, the fam-ily doctor may offer other solutions including surgery. However, despite greater social awareness, mental illness inhabits a separate medical and social sphere.

The recognition, help-seeking, and management of psychiatric phenomena (and neurological) have long been impeded or highly influenced by cultural factors, shaped as they are, by the knowledge, beliefs, and values of the individual and his or her community. The persistence of depression and anxiety symptoms continue to disrupt the possibility of a clear linear connection between an individual's rec-ognition of the problem and when, and from whom, to seek help. Again, such cul-tural factors are not confined to a discussion of ethnicity, even though psychiatric literature in recent years has focussed on minority ethnic disparities. Any group-ing that can be recognised as having values, beliefs, and activities that distinguish them. Social class, gender, and sexual identities have observably different ways of understanding phenomena and acting upon them, and these may play a role in the relationship between trust and medical help-seeking. Here, Kleinman's more sophisticated and complex understanding or schema a healthcare system in which a plurality of often competing belief systems and agencies determine who seeks which kind of help from whom, and when it is sought.

At the less harsh end of mental illness, common mental disorders such as anxi-ety and depression, many people over the course of a lifetime will experience the misery of these disorders which can occur as the result of painful and challenging life events such as bereavement, poor health and disability, unemployment, and so on. Whether these can rightly be called a psychiatric disorder, or as other commentators believe, a normal reaction to life's challenges and sadness provokes considerable and unresolvable controversy (Durà-Vilà, G., Littlewood, R., & Leavey, G. (2013)). This is not to minimise the disruption and distress such problems cause the individual or the economic costs to society. Indeed, many people do not recover from depression and anxiety but experience symptoms intermittently throughout life, and others take their own lives. Nevertheless, however we define these problems, most people affected by depression or anxiety can usually expect to recover spontaneously or through treatment, psychotherapy, or medication.

More intrusively and comprehensively, severe, and enduring psychiatric disorders such as schizophrenia and bipolar disorder typically carry a lifetime of complex problems that undermine most of the life chances that most of us take for granted – such as education, employment, relationships, marriage, and children. In Western societies, people with severe mental illness die prematurely, up to 25 years younger than the general population (Fiorillo & Sartorius, 2021).This mortality rate is often associated with modifiable medical risk factors. In other low- and middle-income countries with scant or no welfare systems and limited healthcare systems in place, life-expectancy for people with mental illness is much less (Hjorthøj et al., 2017). Among populations and communities where resources are scarce, trust is problematic, simply because there is much more at stake for the actors in such environments.

The reason for distinguishing between the different psychiatric diagnoses is not to create a hierarchy of suffering, but rather to argue that there are markedly different levels of health and social impacts on individuals who experience common mental disorders and those who experience severe and enduring mental illnesses such as schizophrenia and bipolar disorder. Individuals with eating disorders and personality disorders may also fit into the more severe and enduring category. However, the concept of trust also requires a reflection regarding severity and impact at several intersections. From the patient's perspective there are phenomenological and ontological matters associated with his or her attempts to grapple with symptoms that intrude into and impose new and often frightening experiences that alter reality, meaning, and behaviour. Even without a severe mental illness, the world can provoke anxieties but the routinisation of daily existence along with a strong dose of cognitive dissonance, most people keep these anxieties at bay. We impose order and structure, and in doing so, unconsciously generate sufficient trust to proceed. The hallucinations and delusional beliefs that feature with severe mental illnesses disrupt the building and maintenance of structures of living, allowing scant space for planning and routinisation in the everyday. Unable to determine what is being experienced and undertaken by whom or what, the capacity of the individual with psychosis to rationalise and to trust is impossible.

That symptoms and behaviours subsumed under the general rubric of a mental illness require a response is an acknowledgement that while they may be a problem for the individual, their family and society more widely, may face challenges of care and control. In its milder form, the risk was posed as a challenge to the family economy; the difficulties posed by incomprehension, the disruption to daily routines, and fulfilling necessary tasks. More seriously and wrongly, mental illness was represented as a physical threat to others.

If trust is conditioned by predictability, the behaviour of person B must be consistent with the characteristics, temperament, beliefs, values, and knowledge that would permit person A to place their trust in person B, treating them in an equitable way that would allow a more favourable outcome. Between them, the relationship provides for relatively smooth and unconscious exchange. However, person A, given particular 'evidence', is more likely to act prejudicially but with mistrust, should they *believe* that person B has a mental illness or has in fact been diagnosed with one. The belief is a lay diagnosis and the other a professional assessment. Both rely on judgements of what is normal or abnormal social behaviour, perhaps based on among other things, the person's history, evidence of previous psychiatric problems, or unusual conduct, and perhaps, a knowledge of the person's culture. Such assessments are contingent on rules and norms found in all societies, frameworks of control and permissibility, determining who, when and where people may behave in a certain way. Examined closely, these rules and the contexts of adherence can appear as absurd, hypocritical, and unjust.

The stranger

The philosopher Charles Taylor states the importance of equal recognition in a 'healthy democratic society' the refusal of which 'can inflict damage on those who are denied it', and that the 'withholding of recognition can be a form of oppression' (Taylor, 2021, p. 31). What constitutes a 'healthy democratic society' is debatable, but by most reasonable definitions this appears currently fragile in most Western nation states. Matters of identity and belonging have been co-opted into the polarising politics of the age. The importance of the concepts of identity and diversity concern issues of equity and justice, and the challenges for developing trust at social, institutional, and personal levels.

Gender dysphoria is the distress experienced by a person due to the incongruence between their own perception of their gender and an incompatible bodily reality. The symptoms associated with gender dysphoria include a persistent cross-gender identification and the desire to be regarded as the other gender (Edition, 2013). Individuals with gender identity dysphoria experience distress because of the sense of being trapped by body parts they don't wish to have, and feelings of inauthenticity of having to *be in* this other body and complying with the particular behavioural norms and dress codes of dress associated with the undesirable identity. Not a mental disorder in itself, gender dysphoria is associated with a high risk of mental illness, self-harm, and suicidality (Aitken et al., 2016). Thus, in childhood and adolescence they are vulnerable low self-esteem and mood disorders. Evidence suggests that increasing numbers of children and young people presenting to health services with gender dysphoria, many presenting at younger ages. Indeed, in the United Kingdom many people have sought to remove its assessment and clinical management from mental health service where it has been situated in the United Kingdom. Identifying the aetiology for gender dysphoria is difficult. For example, it is often accompanied by other conditions such as autism (or traits that indicate an autistic spectrum disorder) (Leavey et al., 2020). Limited public knowledge and perceived clinical uncertainty about how to deal with gender identity has created a challenging environment for those who seek treatment and the services that provide it. Strongly disapproving and sceptical attitudes among the general public, often promoted by religious and conservative forces that incorporate gender (and other identity) issues into cultural antagonisms, feed into the anxieties of parents and families. Service access can be difficult with long delays to be assessed.

Clinicians find themselves caught between commonly competing demands and anxieties of young people and their parents, public and political attitudes, the media, and sometimes, service commissioners. The Tavistock clinic in London, which provided gender-identity services became embroiled in a legal battle concerning the use of puberty blockers (Cass, 2022). At the centre of this dispute was an 'affirmative approach' which appears to accept the young person's expressed gender identity as the basis for treatment. The service's detractors argued that this ready acceptance young person overshadowed and obstructed further exploration that the gender dysphoria might be explained by neurodiversity and/or other complex psychosocial needs, such as those related to childhood trauma. Thus, the argument goes, clinicians within gender dysphoria services may be unwittingly treating the psychosocial expression of a distress, the origins of which lie elsewhere. An affirmative approach sets young people on a pathway towards cross-sex hormones and ultimately, surgical intervention. In accepting the young patients' explanatory models and narratives of distress, as this argument suggests, places skilled and intelligent clinicians in the category of useful dupes or ideologically captured. In battles for identity recognition, the terrain tends to be complex.

Various studies that examined the experiences of individuals accessing specialist gender services highlight the long and complicated pathways in gaining access (Lehmann et al., 2021; Lykens et al., 2018). When they finally do, they describe having to conform to a dominant transgender narrative and presentation before their healthcare needs can be addressed. Thus, non-binary and gender queer patients describe their identities and needs to be dissonant to the clinical models of what an acceptable gender dysphoria patient should be. Obtaining access and treatment can often require the non-binary or queer individual to appropriate a binary identity.

In our own study of non-binary patients and help-seeking (Lehmann et al., 2021), we used Goffman's theory on impression management, which emphasises human flexibility and reflexiveness in the enactment of various and distinct roles that are consonant with context and task. We sought explore the strategies used by non-binary patients to overcome perceived barriers to the access of gender identity services. Key to such strategies was the belief that their gender identity needed to be consistent and stable, rather than fluctuating between identities, or rather how an identity might be represented and perceived by others. Several participants described a 'frontstage' presentation of a stable identity designed to reassure staff despite when the potential for an irreversible treatment was being decided, even when the patient's sense of identity was not concretely fixed. While this pretence served a function for both participants and staff, it unfortunately did not address underlying issues that may have required further therapeutic exploration. While preparing for 'frontstage' clinical consultations they manufactured what they considered an idealised version of their true gender, that is, outwardly binary, either ultra-feminine or ultra-masculine ways. These performative aspects of gender dysphoria patients' help-seeking reveal much more vividly than perhaps other 'medical' conditions, medical mistrust of people who seek intervention, a mistrust partly explained by resource rationing and highly governed by normative and non-normative stereotypes.

Culture and recognition

Like most cultural rules, there are degrees of flexibility and fluidity relating to whom they should apply, for example, or how long they can be sustained. Sending young children to beg sweets from neighbours and strangers would be unthinkable at any other time of the year other than Halloween – similarly, the riotous behaviours at Diwali or Purim. However, such behaviours described as rites of reversal or symbolic inversion (Shepherd & Babcock, 1978), the purpose of which is a controlled transgression – 'letting off steam' rather than promoting a plausible alternative lifestyle. Helman (2007, p. 247) makes the point that in situations of controlled abnormality such as war where fundamentally powerful taboos against killing and other atrocities are suspended temporarily, after which time people are expected to return to 'normality' as best they can. The fluidity of societal norms related to what is considered abnormal are exemplified by shifting attitudes and legislation on sexuality, gender, and drug use.

Lay assessment of normality may rest on social cues and indicators such dress, hygiene, facial expression, and language. Crucially, while the individual's behaviour should be consonant with the context and circumstances, it should also be appropriate to their personal history and characteristics – that is, to what their family and peers have come to expect. For others not so well acquainted, does the person's behaviour conform to age, sex, education, job, culture, and so on.[3] Thus, people will make their own judgement about whether a person is mad or bad, unless perhaps they happen to be a family member, but this matters little since the response by the public is often the same, that is, avoidance. Lay people can and do make incorrect and damaging assessments of others. Specialist professional training and assessment should be a counterweight to lay misappraisal.

Psychiatry must make its own determination about a person's insight and motivations in circumstances of apparent abnormal social behaviour. In most medical diagnoses, disorder is measured by various observable and generally unambiguous biological indicators. Such indicators of health and wellbeing are not available to psychiatrists. A mentally disturbed and highly irate individual may well have a high blood pressure but that is insufficient to confirm a psychiatric diagnosis. While the body of knowledge on genetic variation and treatment is growing rapidly, there remain no clear markers for schizophrenia despite the known high heritability of this challenging disorder. While recent studies demonstrate promising advances in this area, early identification and treatments are a long way off (Singh et al., 2022).

In any case, a constant barrier to accurate psychiatric diagnostic methods is that the indicators of abnormality do not conform to neat a binary of positives and negatives. Rather, they are generally found on a wide continuum of human behaviours, not just between cultures but within the same culture. Snake handling and glossolalia might be unusual among Episcopalians and metropolitan intellectual elites, and while they may be commonly perceived as strange, at best, they have their place in various minority churches and communities. The immense heterogeneity of human beliefs and behaviours add to the unreliability of an easy determination of abnormality. While schizophrenia is characterised by delusional ideas, how should we react to surveys which regularly reveal that more than two-thirds of Americans believe in angels and that spiritual energy may emerge from physical entities such as plants, rivers, or crystals.[4] Belief in alien visitation and the personal experience of alien abduction is held by 1% of the population, a similar proportion of clinically diagnosed schizophrenia. It is significant that psychotic experiences are also commonly reported among non-clinical populations. Thus, the Dunedin cohort study which examined the data of children through to adulthood found that adolescents commonly endorsed symptoms (abnormal beliefs and hallucinations) typical of a psychotic disorder. While these children appear to have had a higher risk of schizophrenia, the outcome was not inevitable. Other surveys note the presence of delusions and hallucinations among otherwise ordinary non-clinical populations (Stip & Letourneau, 2009).

It has been hypothesised that the distribution of psychotic experiences in a population indicates a phenomenological continuum across clinical and non-clinical populations, ranging from intense, clinically significant psychotic symptoms to trait-like dispositions, and more subtle psychotic-like experiences. Some researchers have suggested that clinical and non-clinical psychotic experiences can be observed as an extended psychosis phenotype, with similar genetic, cognitive, and psychosocial psychopathological features (van Os et al., 2009).[5]

Psychiatry and its discontents

While a medicalised social control argument maybe unconvincing, suspicions that medicine, particularly psychiatry is appropriating natural or normal aspects of life, started with the use of tranquillisers to manage stress and anxiety, predominantly supplied to women and 'housewives', until their addictive qualities became publicly known. Later in the 1990s, something of a prescribing and cultural revolution occurred with the advent of Selective Serotonin Reuptake Inhibitors (SSRI), which promised to have few of the difficult side effects of the tricyclic antidepressant medication and might be the cure for human misery. The supply and demand for SSRIs has never plateaued since their introduction despite evidence that they are inappropriate for people with major depression and possibly harmful for various demographic sectors. Despite widespread use they seem to have had no impact in reducing suicide rates anywhere but then, neither has increased affluence in Western societies, leading to a view that the origins of, and preventative solutions to, depression may reside in social relations rather than body chemistry. Problematically for progressive social policy in modern economies, 'individual fixes' based on individualist ideologies are an easier sell than restructuring social goals and relationships. Accordingly, it is more economically profitable to suppress symptoms of distress than eradicate their causes.

To date, there have been numerous studies on the medicalisation of sadness, loneliness, shyness, sexual dysfunction, and social anxiety (Bandini, 2015; Durà-Vilà et al., 2013; Horwitz & Wakefield, 2007). To a range of addictions related to alcohol and substance misuse, sexual promiscuity, and internet use are now regarded as territory for psychiatry and designated as psychiatric conditions under the various editions of the DSM. Davis suggests that studies related to medicalisation 'generally recognise or presuppose a boundary between normal and expectable experience and a chronic and debilitating condition' (Davis, 2010, p. 227). However, of interest to academic observers and social commentators alike, is a possible lowering in recent years of the 'public' threshold for tolerance of different emotional and psychological 'conditions' and their consequent lay recognition as a problem requiring treatment.

The rise in antidepressants in Western countries over the past decade is striking, especially for young people (Bachmann et al., 2016; Jack et al., 2020), begging various questions about what is driving these increases. First, are more people using antidepressants because they are too readily prescribed by physicians or because, similar to the over-prescription of antibiotics, are patients now culturally conditioned to expect them through increasing awareness and media conversation about 'mental health'? An area that was once considered shameful and off-limits by most people has developed an interesting level of acceptability within the social discourses of young people. Biographical revelations by high-profile role models such as musicians, members of the British royal family, and media celebrities create a more accommodating and non-judgemental social ambience in which the general population can reveal their own 'struggles with mental health'. However, these revelations are predominantly related to common mental disorders and never, as far as one knows, related to severe and enduring mental illnesses such as schizophrenia or bipolar disorder for which the prevalence remains stable. Depression, it would appear, appears somewhat de-stigmatised while schizophrenia remains unacceptable. Market research on the use of internet-based educational tools for mental illness suggests that fears about psychosis would reduce the numbers of people using these sites (Henderson, 2023).

That such shifts (or not) are culturally shaped appears to be supported by the content analysis of stigmatising of mental illnesses within newspaper articles in

England over an eight-year period (Hildersley et al., 2020). Importantly, anti-stigma, and/or mental health literacy campaigns, commonly focus on common mental disorders or are pitched at a level of vague generality, lacking in any description about particular disorders – the messaging in such campaigns is about 'mental health problems'. It has also been observed that these campaigns also tend to expand the concept of mental illness to include stress and grief. Between 2009 and 2019, the proportion of people endorsing stress as a mental illness rose by 10%, with a similar increase for grief. These findings provide further evidence of a creeping medicalisation of normal human experience but not that these are being driven by the psychiatric profession. Nevertheless, despite criticism of Western biomedicine, the medical profession has maintained its place as a dominant provider of healthcare, and it is hard to envisage its decline. But, behind the more observed, measured, and evaluated professional healthcare system exists an unnoticed complex web of healthcare activity by people 'in the community'.

The end of misery

Similarly, ordinary human stress and unhappiness, arising from our environment and social relationships are increasingly treated with antidepressants, sedatives, and anxiolytics. The demand for instant 'fixes' for our troubles has grown exponentially. Another critique of medicine, and psychiatry especially, is that it extends beyond the clinical management of 'natural' problems of life and challenging experiences, and into the social control of what might be more appropriately considered as deviant behaviour. For psychiatry, these raise difficult questions about legitimacy, jurisdiction and who benefits – are psychiatric activities in support of the patient or is the true client the state, operating in its own interests within boundaries of its choosing?

We can trace some of this critique to Parsons' notion of the 'sick role', a functionalist perspective on what he considered a societal need to regulate illness in the same way that other forms of deviancy need to be controlled. By adopting the 'sick role' and surrendering to the diagnosis and advice of the doctor, the patient is excused from normal duties (and exculpated from responsibility for the illness), but strives to 'get better', a contractual arrangement that maintains order. Parsons' sick role, was highly criticised for what was a rather cynical view of both patients' needs and an obvious distortion of clinical utility – not just the relevance and usefulness of an intervention in medicine but the totality of benefits each party derives (Beutler & Howard, 1998).

Nevertheless, some of Parsons' ideas related to the sick role resonate with matters of the patient–doctor relationship. First the state's and organisational management of sickness (and welfare) with a clearly designated power imbalance that may undermine medical claims of neutrality: that doctors may not be working in the best interests of the patient but rather the employer and/or the state. In the United Kingdom and elsewhere, as economic pressures mount on welfare systems there is a renewed muscularity in 'clamping down' on so-called 'free-riders'(Øverland et al., 2008).[6] Second, Parsons' conceptualisation of the patient adopting a 'role', while apparently cynical, may nevertheless assist us in thinking about the performative aspects of the doctor–patient role, particularly in relation to the relatively invisible disorders and disabilities which rely heavily, if not exclusively, on what the patient can, or wishes to, describe. Or in the case of a parent escorting a child to the doctor, describing symptoms or behaviours of 'something not quite right' that are observed.

All parties must consider what is at stake in this encounter. The patient (or family) must seek to convince that there is a medical need and that it can be met in some vague way by the doctor. Although in some cases, patients will have a very specific intervention in mind. The doctor must weigh up the evidence presented, again in the absence of any biological correlates. While objective evidence of a diagnosable mental illness is desirable, the consultation is primarily conducted subjectively; the explanation of complex feelings and non-normative behaviours that may make little sense to the patient (and/or the patient's family), and are met with a high degree of interpretability by primary care doctors who commonly lack confidence and training in dealing with mental illness (Docherty, 1997). Both parties are formally engaged in making sense of phenomena expressed, not just in words but also conveyed by appearance in dress and bodily expression, eye contact, and affect in speech. Into this space too both bring their cultural backgrounds, potentially quite different worlds of experience and education, which are often tacit but salient. Doctors may attempt a determination of a mental health problem using strict diagnostic criteria but are likely also to seek some contextual and causal explanations such as work, stress, alcohol use, relationship problems, and so forth. Patients may have a relatively clear view of what they want from these encounters. That they seek help from a doctor at all indicates an explanatory model that aligns with an understanding of what the doctor can offer, which may be hospitalisation, pharmaceutical treatment, or a talking therapy.

In as much as the patient's interpretation of the symptoms and feelings corresponds with those of the doctor's, we might assume that the patient trusts the physician's assessment; where their respective appraisals of illness and/or treatment differ, trust in the doctor may be diminished. But it is also the case that in many patient–doctor consultations there are no diagnosable problems, at least problems with a biological origin, or that the problems are insignificantly alarming to require medical assistance. The somatic presentation may mask various underlying emotional problems that are the genuine reason for the clinical consultation but cannot be articulated for whatever reason. Mechanic (1980, p. 206) referring to Balint's view of the masked clinical consultation, suggests that such complaints may be a pathway to achieving help, but also an oblique way of obtaining reassurance and support in a socially acceptable way. This is common when it is difficult to seek help for the underlying (true) reason without revealing 'weaknesses and vulnerabilities contrary to expected and learned behaviour patterns'. Mechanic additionally suggests that while a somatic presentation may be instrumental for people who lack psychologic literacy, even those who are able to express themselves psychologically, may avoid doing so to avoid being regarded as hypochondriacal. Much of what is unspoken and/or unconscious in the patient–doctor negotiation, is in Bourdieu's terms, establishing 'the rules of the game' – that is, what can the doctor be trusted to accept, and how the doctor will respond to psychological/emotional concerns of the patient. At times, the rules of the game are not always clear, particularly so when different actors in the negotiated space of the consultation differ in terms of the diagnosis and desired outcome.

In a study of patient suicide and consultations with family doctors, families were distressed when physicians were easily deceived according to the relative's narrative, by the light-hearted and entirely false presentation provided by patients who shortly afterwards, took their own lives (Leavey et al., 2016, 2017). I have described these encounters as 'contests', between the patient and other family members, provoking frustration and resentment. In the same study, participants stated that doctors can often misinterpret, or possibly ignore, patient communication. From the other side of the clinical encounter, family doctors draw on various factors to consider the likely veracity of patients' claims, and seldom acknowledged, is that demographic and other contextual stereotypes may inform clinical judgement. Thus, because the evidence tells us that most non-fatal suicide attempts are carried out by women and that completed suicides are overwhelmingly by men, we noted that primary care physicians were less likely to provide follow-up for women who subsequently took their own lives.

Moreover, we noted that many of the General Practitioners in deprived inner-city areas discussed their health care in the midst of community problems of drug abuse and gang violence. They reported feeling pressurised by the demand for sick notes and psychiatric medication, often for illegal reasons. In such circumstance GPs develop a mistrust of patients who present as having social problems which tend to overshadow their medical problems, producing morally tinged medical judgements. These judgements are also determined by a GP's role and responsibility as a budget-holder of public funds. Stereotyping may guide the judgement. Thus, again noted in discussions with GPs, the questions that may arise in assessing patient needs are prefaced by queries about the authenticity of the person's illness and their motivation in seeking help – are they really ill or in need of medication for recreational use or to obtain welfare benefits.

Moreover, many GPs lack training in the management of mental illness. Given the commonality of depression, the ability to ascertain and treat patient suicidality is a challenge to medical competence and confidence. If most suicidal patients do not readily disclose their suicidality, it is believed that brief standardised screening questions might be helpful. However, many GPs remain unconvinced, considering this as counterproductive, provoking defensiveness among patients and a barrier to therapeutic engagement or undermining their skills in some way. But in many respects, suicide remains unpredictable because, despite the known risk factors there is no 'obvious suicidal patient' in terms of the patient characteristics, social contexts, and presenting problems. Of course, part of the unspoken contract between patient and doctor is that patients will act in good faith and provide truthful responses, but it is in this contest that the lines get blurred, only made clearer if the doctor has a long connection with the patient. The unpredictability may arise for example through an individual's somatic presentations which exclude any discussion of psychiatric complaints or through regular attendance at the practice for routine complaints. Doctors reported astonishment and grief when older patients managing chronic conditions, highly regarded for stoicism, later take their own lives. Unlike patients who are noted to have 'social problems', such patients are trusted by doctors because of their familiarity and reliability. There are no concerns about their motivation in seeking health care. In other cases, doctors are deeply affected by patient suicide when they feel that a long-standing trust has been breached by deception.

Trust and shared health beliefs

In addition to recognising the presence of a problem which effects their health and wellbeing that requires external help, those seeking help from a medical practitioner must first be able to define its nature in terms that are consonant with a medical model or framework. Where there is dissonance between the patient's and the practitioner's assessment of the problem, the potential for treatment and adherence is considerably limited. In this sense, trust can only emerge between patient and doctor if they have a shared understanding of the nature and source of the problem or, even where the patient's initial view of things differs from that of the doctor, the former accedes to the latter's knowledge and diagnosis. In situations where there is cultural variation in health beliefs, the development of trust between healthcare professionals and patients, can be problematic. This kind of disjunction is mostly associated with ethnicity and multi-ethnic societies, but not exclusively so. Importantly though, the challenge of trust-building in healthcare is particularly prominent in the contested world of minority ethnic communities, psychiatric disorders, and treatment.

There is considerable variation in the social or cultural acceptability of certain bodily complaints, and in some cases, the nature and site of such complaints within different groups. Indeed, much of the medical sociological and anthropology literature describes how bodily complaints and pain are expressed by various cultural groups, from stoicism to almost unbearable anxiety (Tsai et al., 2004; Varela et al., 2004; Zola, 1966). The apparent high prevalence of somatisation in non-Western cultures has been associated with low levels of interoceptive awareness – the sensitivity to bodily changes, is noted among many non-Western populations (Ma-Kellams, 2014). In various Asian cultures emotional experiences are often located within bodily organs and described in these terms (Good & Good, 1980; Kleinman, 1981). However, even in Western societies, the expression of emotional states through location in body parts has a long tradition; for example, 'brokenhearted', 'heart-sinking', and 'gut-wrenching'. Thus, cultural variation in somatic complaints may be overstated according to the findings from a WHO study (Gureje et al., 1997) which noted few differences in the frequency of unexplained somatic symptoms related to geography or level of economic development. Nevertheless, the study also showed that somatising patients perceive their health more negatively, and consequently, have an elevated risk of comorbid depression and generalised anxiety disorder.

However, even when (or perhaps because) patients have a reasonable grasp of psychological literacy, they may be more assertive about their treatment preferences in the clinical encounter. In our study of young people and mental health, a commonly expressed view was that antidepressant or anxiolytic medication were too easily used by doctors as a way of dismissing the patient, and not providing consultation space to understand what the 'real' underlying causes and needs might be (Corry & Leavey, 2017). These and other aspects of the health system undermine the medicalisation argument that positions medicine as a tool at the disposal of the state in the control of 'deviance'. Thus, patients cannot be perceived as passive victims or dupes. As consumers, they can sift through the evidence and weigh this against personal previous experiences and those of other people in their network. Increasingly, people will also seek advice and guidance from internet sources which are easily accessible, have no geographical boundaries, and are usually privacy preserving, which obviates the stigma in help-seeking for emotional and psychological problems. Increasingly too, the internet is a platform for self-initiated and directed, low-intensity mental health support. Others may facilitate screening and decision-making tools to direct individuals appropriately to health professionals (Kauer et al., 2014). Although attractive to services there is scant evidence on the effectiveness of these platforms and tools, and little is known about how individuals assess the trustworthiness of this information or their behaviour in scepticism of, or adherence to internet-based information, leaving some gaps in our understanding of trust behaviour in these media. Nevertheless, the volume of traffic on health internet sites is evidence of some degree of patient autonomy and agency.

Secondly, the medical control of deviance implies the connivance of physicians, that they too are unconscious dupes of the system. Moreover, a deviance control theory neglects the complex, contextual differences between medical systems that are the products of the socio-economic and cultural systems in which they are based. To consider trust in these systems, an analysis is required of medicine's financial basis, physician funding, and political power – where is the doctor's place within the power structure and who pays their salaries? Thus, the autonomy of doctors in the United States compared to their UK counterparts are substantially different because of the distinctive funding sources. Additionally, while both are systems are highly regulated, the NHS has more controls over what medication and treatments can be offered; for example, the attempt to constrain the prescribing habits of family doctors through the central guidance of a National Institute for Health and Care Excellence. International efforts by the WHO and Centre for Disease Control have had chequered success in reducing the flow of antimicrobial medicines, painkillers, and antidepressants (Dowell et al., 2016; Kendrick, 2021; Organization, 2014).

Mistrust or paranoia

Mistrust (like trust) can assume multiple forms in how it is operationalised and practiced. Unlike trust, mistrust as a concept and as attitude and behaviour, has attracted less academic attention from medical sociologists, or in the trust literature, more generally. Psychiatry, for reasons we will explore, may have more to say about mistrust. Whereas most theories of trust conceptualise it as having an implicit acceptance of vulnerability, mistrust is directed towards the actual or perceived vulnerability with the purpose of reducing the threat or minimising its impact if it can't be avoided. Thus, to mistrust is a preparation for action where possible, and to strategise given a range of options. To act with mistrust towards others or an institution, at least rationally, one acts upon available evidence, directly or indirectly conveyed by personal experience or that of others. The information may be correct or incorrectly conveyed as lies, or perhaps misinterpretation. The information may be true but the information provider unreliable or untrustworthy. Thus, the source and motivations of the information provider are worth considering too. Like the 'boy who cried wolf', those who continue to provide faulty information that later proves false will have a diminishing level of credibility and effect.

However, distinguishing pathological paranoid symptoms from the often-overwhelming fears and anxieties that are held by individuals and groups universally is problematic. The world has always been dangerous and the relatively recent universal awareness of environmental disasters through climate change has only served to intensify fears and provoke a blossoming of conspiracy theories, claims, and counterclaims. Although we may not live in a conflict zone where violence is prevalent, many people work (or play) in highly competitive sectors in which all manner of harmful behaviours are exhibited and experienced, including threats to self-esteem and sanity. It is estimated that between 10% and 15% of general population experience paranoid beliefs. Indeed, a large British survey of over 8,000 people, excluding people with a probable psychosis showed that 20% of the sample believed that people were against them at times, and 10% believed that other people had deliberately acted to harm them (Johns et al., 2004). Again, it is noted that 1% to 3%, approximately, of the non-clinical population experience delusions at a level of severity that may be comparable to people with a psychotic illness and 5% to 6% experience delusions of less severity, but still associated with social and emotional difficulties (Freeman, 2007).

Freeman makes a strong case for a consideration of 'paranoid' or persecutory beliefs in the general population rather than solely a clinical population, suggesting that paranoid thoughts may be an appropriate strategy in dealing with the threats of others but may become excessive in the same way that anxious thoughts can overwhelm some people. If there is an overlap in the content of beliefs in clinical and non-clinical populations, it is possible that a specific focus on the former only serves as a confirmatory bias, rather than a clear distinguishing dimension. It is likely that particular ideological belief systems, whether political or religious, that appear to be extreme or highly unusual, will clash with those that sit outside the normative belief system of health care professionals. Deciding what is a sincerely held belief, a delusion or a manipulative confidence trick is the challenge in many psychiatric cases. In some situations, the views of the public and psychiatry may not differ too much and may not be a significant epistemological task. For example, religious cults adherents are convinced by charismatic leaders to adopt 'dooms-day' persecutory beliefs and to undertake highly dangerous and morally dubious behaviours in support of these, mostly for the perverse gratification of the leaders. However, Western healthcare systems, not just psychiatric services, are regularly confronted by faith groups and individuals whose beliefs on everything from birth delivery and blood transfusion to vaccines and spirit possession, provoke disso-nance and mutual mistrust. Regardless of problematic beliefs people from minority ethnic and migrant backgrounds have worse physical and mental health outcomes than their indigenous white equivalents. The COVID 19 pandemic found them to be at higher risk of the illness and of dying (Wang et al., 2021).

While some of the personal risk of mental disorders is inherited, and some disorders such as schizophrenia, have more heritability than others, much of the vulnerability is shaped by factors related to social and family environments that individuals are born into and over which they have no control. These same envi-ronments produce interpersonal relationships, experiences, and events that shape our mental health and form our understanding of how to manage and cope with such problems as they arise. Into this complex mix, personality, the product of nature and nurture, plays a role too. While genetics offer hope in changing the heritability to illness, cures and transformations remain a distant aspiration. This leaves us with a focus on the social and environmental factors that provoke vul-nerability and undermine the various dimensions of trust that support our mental health and wellbeing; these factors must also be examined in how they accom-modate our needs when symptoms arise, and mental health deteriorates. In this way, the concept of trust is related to mental health over the life course, childhood and parenting, adversities, and the emergence of mental illness, help-seeking, and social support.

Notes

1 Szasz (P51) also argues that in a previous age that confronted with a person without any obvious bodily illness there was a tendency to think that such a person ought to submit 'to the ministrations of either medicine or theology' but now, psychiatry has replaced theology – a view also held by Charles Taylor, affirming the view of psychotherapists and psychiatrists as modern-day priests.
2 A fascinating and highly publicised study that would be unlikely to ever obtain ethical approval from current university or hospital ethics committees. The study, however, raises many questions about the legitimacy of the methods used by the pseudo-patients, and the claims and conclusions made by Rosenham. For example, had the pseudo-pa-tients acted 'normally' following admission, it would be expected that 'normal' people would have protested their sanity and demanded to be released right away. This never happened.

3 Asserting the doctrine of the divine right of kings in 17th-century England might have been regarded as foolish but not a sign of insanity, while the latter would certainly be more likely in the 21st century.

4 AP-NORC Center for Public Affairs Research (July 2023). 'Belief in angels and heaven is more common than belief in the devil or hell'. https://apnorc.org/projects/belief-in-angels-and-heaven-is-more-common-than-belief-in-the-devil-or-hell/

5 In this meta-analysis, some of the risk factors for psychosis showed associations with developmental stage, social adversity in childhood, drug use, and migrant status. Van Os and colleagues also noted between 75% and 90%, approximately, of developmental psychotic experiences may be transitory. However, that the transitory developmental expression of psychosis subsequently develops into clinically relevant problems, depending on environmental and other exposures.

6 UK policy introduced in 2010 under Work Capability Assessment was independently associated with an increase in suicides and mental health problems. However, in contradiction of medical bias towards the state, much of the antipathy and resistance to the processes and findings of the WCCA came from the medical profession. who

References

Aitken, M., VanderLaan, D. P., Wasserman, L., Stojanovski, S., & Zucker, K. J. (2016). Self-harm and suicidality in children referred for gender dysphoria. *Journal of the American Academy of Child & Adolescent Psychiatry, 55*(6), 513–520. https://doi.org/10.1016/j.jaac.2016.04.001

Arendt, H. (1970). *On violence.* Harcourt.

Bachmann, C. J., Aagaard, L., Burcu, M., Glaeske, G., Kalverdijk, L. J., Petersen, I., Schuiling-Veninga, C. C., Wijlaars, L., Zito, J. M., & Hoffmann, F. (2016). Trends and patterns of antidepressant use in children and adolescents from five western countries, 2005-2012. *Eur Neuropsychopharmacol, 26*(3), 411–419. https://doi.org/10.1016/j.euroneuro.2016.02.001

Bandini, J. (2015). The medicalization of bereavement: (Ab)normal grief in the DSM-5. *Death Studies, 39*(6), 347–352. https://doi.org/10.1080/07481187.2014.951498

Beutler, L. E., & Howard, K. I. (1998). Clinical utility research: An introduction. *Journal of Clinical Psychology, 54*(3), 297–301. https://doi.org/10.1002/(sici)1097-4679(199804)54:3<297::aid-jclp1>3.0.co;2-n

Bracken, P., & Thomas, P. (2010). From Szasz to Foucault: On the role of critical psychiatry. *Philosophy, Psychiatry, and Psychology, 17*(3), 219–228.

Cass, H. (2022). *Independent review of gender identity services for children and young people: Interim report.* NHS England, London.

Corry, D. A., & Leavey, G. (2017). Adolescent trust and primary care: Help-seeking for emotional and psychological difficulties. *Journal of Adolescence, 54*, 1–8. https://doi.org/10.1016/j.adolescence.2016.11.003

Davis, J. E. (2010). Medicalization, social control, and the relief of suffering. In W. C. Cockerham (Ed.), *The Blackwell companion to medical sociology* (pp. 211–241). Wiley.

Docherty, J. P. (1997). Barriers to the diagnosis of depression in primary care. *Journal of Clinical Psychiatry, 58*(1), 5–10.

Dowell, D., Haegerich, T. M., & Chou, R. (2016). CDC guideline for prescribing opioids for chronic pain—United States, 2016. *JAMA, 315*(15), 1624–1645. https://doi.org/10.1001/jama.2016.1464

Durà-Vilà, G., Littlewood, R., & Leavey, G. (2013). Depression and the medicalization of sadness: Conceptualization and recommended help-seeking. *International Journal of Social Psychiatry, 59*(2), 165–175. https://doi.org/10.1177/0020764011430037

Edition, F. (2013). Diagnostic and statistical manual of mental disorders. *American Psychiatric Association, 21*(21), 591–643.

Fiorillo, A., & Sartorius, N. (2021). Mortality gap and physical comorbidity of people with severe mental disorders: The public health scandal. *Annals of General Psychiatry, 20*(1), 52. https://doi.org/10.1186/s12991-021-00374-y

Freeman, D. (2007). Suspicious minds: The psychology of persecutory delusions. *Clinical Psychology Review, 27*(4), 425–457. https://doi.org/10.1016/j.cpr.2006.10.004

Giddens, A. (1991). *Modernity and self-identity: Self and society in the late modern age.* Polity Press.

Good, B. J., & Good, M. J. D. (1980). The meaning of symptoms: A cultural hermeneutic model for clinical practice. In L. Eisenberg, Kleinman, A. (Eds.), *The relevance of social science for medicine* (pp. 165–196). Springer.

Gureje, O., Simon, G. E., Ustun, T. B., & Goldberg, D. P. (1997). Somatization in cross-cultural perspective: A world health organization study in primary care. *American Journal of Psychiatry, 154*(7), 989–995. https://doi.org/10.1176/ajp.154.7.989

Helman, C. (2007). *Culture, health and illness, fifth edition.* CRC Press.

Henderson, C. (2023). Challenges in improving mental health literacy at population level. *World Psychiatry, 22*(3), 392–393. https://doi.org/10.1002/wps.21115

Hildersley, R., Potts, L., Anderson, C., & Henderson, C. (2020). Improvement for most, but not all: Changes in newspaper coverage of mental illness from 2008 to 2019 in England. *Epidemiology and Psychiatric Sciences, 29*, e177. https://doi.org/10.1017/s204579602000089x

Hjorthøj, C., Stürup, A. E., McGrath, J. J., & Nordentoft, M. (2017). Years of potential life lost and life expectancy in schizophrenia: A systematic review and meta-analysis. *The Lancet Psychiatry, 4*(4), 295–301. https://doi.org/10.1016/S2215-0366(17)30078-0

Horwitz, A. V., & Wakefield, J. C. (2007). *The loss of sadness: How psychiatry transformed normal sorrow into depressive disorder.* Oxford University Press.

Jack, R. H., Hollis, C., Coupland, C., Morriss, R., Knaggs, R. D., Butler, D., Cipriani, A., Cortese, S., & Hippisley-Cox, J. (2020). Incidence and prevalence of primary care antidepressant prescribing in children and young people in England, 1998–2017: A population-based cohort study. *PLOS Medicine, 17*(7), e1003215. https://doi.org/10.1371/journal.pmed.1003215

Johns, L. C., Cannon, M., Singleton, N., Murray, R. M., Farrell, M., Brugha, T., Bebbington, P., Jenkins, R., & Meltzer, H. (2004). Prevalence and correlates of self-reported psychotic symptoms in the British population. *The British Journal of Psychiatry, 185*(4), 298–305.

Kauer, S. D., Mangan, C., & Sanci, L. (2014). Do online mental health services improve help-seeking for young people? A systematic review. *Journal of Medical Internet Research, 16*(3), e66. https://doi.org/10.2196/jmir.3103

Kendrick, T. (2021). Strategies to reduce use of antidepressants. *British Journal of Clinical Pharmacology, 87*(1), 23–33. https://doi.org/10.1111/bcp.14475

King, M., Smith, G., & Bartlett, A. (2004). Treatments of homosexuality in Britain since The 1950s–an oral history: The experience of professionals. *BMJ, 328*(7437), 429. https://doi.org/10.1136/bmj.37984.496725.EE

Kleinman, A. (1981). *Patients and healers in the context of culture; an exploration of the borderland between, anthropology, medicine and psychiatry.* University of California Press.

Leavey, G., Lehmann, K., McKenna, H., & Rosato, M. (2020). Autism trait prevalence in treatment seeking adolescents and adults attending specialist gender services. *European Psychiatry, 63*(1), e23, Article e23. https://doi.org/10.1192/j.eurpsy.2020.23

Leavey, G., Mallon, S., Rondon-Sulbaran, J., Galway, K., Rosato, M., & Hughes, L. (2017). The failure of suicide prevention in primary care: Family and GP perspectives – a qualitative study. *BMC Psychiatry, 17*(1), 369. https://doi.org/10.1186/s12888-017-1508-7

Leavey, G., Rosato, M., Galway, K., Hughes, L., Mallon, S., & Rondon, J. (2016). Patterns and predictors of help seeking contacts with health services and general practice detection of suicidality. *BMC Psychiatry*, *16*(1), 120.

Lehmann, K., Rosato, M., McKenna, H., & Leavey, G. (2021). Dramaturgical accounts of transgender individuals: Impression management in the presentation of self to specialist gender services. *Archives of Sexual Behavior*, *50*(8), 3539–3549. https://doi.org/10.1007/s10508-021-02028-2

Lykens, J. E., LeBlanc, A. J., & Bockting, W. O. (2018). Healthcare experiences among young adults who identify as genderqueer or nonbinary. *LGBT Health*, *5*(3), 191–196.

Ma-Kellams, C. (2014). Cross-cultural differences in somatic awareness and interoceptive accuracy: A review of the literature and directions for future research [Review]. *Frontiers in Psychology*, *5*. https://doi.org/10.3389/fpsyg.2014.01379

Mechanic, D. (1980). The presentation of bodily complaints. In D. Mechanic (Ed.), *Readings in medical sociology* The Free Press.

Organization, W. H. (2014). *Antimicrobial resistance: Global report on surveillance*. World Health Organization.

Øverland, S., Glozier, N., Henderson, M., Mæland, J. G., Hotopf, M., & Mykletun, A. (2008). Health status before, during and after disability pension award: The Hordaland Health Study (HUSK). *Occupational and Environmental Medicine*, *65*(11), 769–773. https://doi.org/10.1136/oem.2007.037861

Patel, V., Chisholm, D., Parikh, R., Charlson, F. J., Degenhardt, L., Dua, T., Ferrari, A. J., Hyman, S., Laxminarayan, R., Levin, C., Lund, C., Medina Mora, M. E., Petersen, I., Scott, J., Shidhaye, R., Vijayakumar, L., Thornicroft, G., & Whiteford, H. (2016). Addressing the burden of mental, neurological, and substance use disorders: Key messages from disease control priorities, 3rd edition. *Lancet*, *387*(10028), 1672–1685. https://doi.org/10.1016/s0140-6736(15)00390-6

Porter, R. (1997). *The greatest benefit to mankind: A medical history of humanity from antiquity to the present*. Fontana Press.

Scull, A. (2019). *Psychiatry and its discontents*. University of California.

Scull, A. T. (1977). Madness and segregative control: The rise of the insane asylum. *Social Problems*, *24*(3), 337–351.

Shepherd, G., & Babcock, B. A. (1978). The reversible world: Symbolic inversion in art and society.

Singh, T., Poterba, T., Curtis, D., Akil, H., Al Eissa, M., Barchas, J. D., Bass, N., Bigdeli, T. B., Breen, G., Bromet, E. J., Buckley, P. F., Bunney, W. E., Bybjerg-Grauholm, J., Byerley, W. F., Chapman, S. B., Chen, W. J., Churchhouse, C., Craddock, N., Cusick, C. M., … Daly, M. J. (2022). Rare coding variants in ten genes confer substantial risk for schizophrenia. *Nature*, *604*(7906), 509–516. https://doi.org/10.1038/s41586-022-04556-w

Stip, E., & Letourneau, G. (2009). Psychotic symptoms as a continuum between normality and pathology. *The Canadian Journal of Psychiatry*, *54*(3), 141–151.

Szasz, T. (1973). *The manufacture of madness*. Paladin.

Taylor, C. (2021). The politics of recognition. In *Campus wars* (pp. 249–263). Routledge.

Tsai, J. L., Simeonova, D. I., & Watanabe, J. T. (2004). Somatic and social: Chinese Americans talk about emotion. *Personality and Social Psychology Bulletin*, *30*(9), 1226–1238. https://doi.org/10.1177/0146167204264014

van Os, J., Linscott, R. J., Myin-Germeys, I., Delespaul, P., & Krabbendam, L. (2009). A systematic review and meta-analysis of the psychosis continuum: Evidence for a psychosis proneness-persistence-impairment model of psychotic disorder. *Psychological Medicine*, *39*(2), 179–195. https://doi.org/10.1017/s0033291708003814

Varela, R. E., Vernberg, E. M., Sanchez-Sosa, J. J., Riveros, A., Mitchell, M., & Mashunkashey, J. (2004). Anxiety reporting and culturally associated interpretation biases and cognitive schemas: A comparison of Mexican, Mexican American, and European American families. *Journal of Clinical Child & Adolescent Psychology*, *33*(2), 237–247. https://doi.org/10.1207/s15374424jccp3302_4

Wang, Q., Xu, R., & Volkow, N. D. (2021). Increased risk of COVID-19 infection and mortality in people with mental disorders: Analysis from electronic health records in the United States. *World Psychiatry, 20*(1), 124–130. https://doi.org/10.1002/wps.20806

Zola, I. K. (1966). Culture and symptoms: An analysis of patients' presenting complaints. *American Sociological Review, 31*, 615–630.

Chapter 8

Structural Dimensions of Mistrust

Familiarity and routinisation are key dimensions in the shaping of trust. The longer we know someone, the deeper our connections with them, the greater the potential for a trusting relationship, and betrayal, of course. Familiarity in the form of ethnicity – defined as having a shared history, geographical origins, language, religion, or cultural norms (Senior & Bhopal, 1994) – plays a role, at least partially, in the determination of trust at an interpersonal and intergroup level. Not to be confused with the highly problematic concept of race,[1] ethnicity is more closely related to self-identity, and thus, may shift over time. Importantly, the absence of shared experience, knowledge, language, and communication, diminishes the opportunities for trust-formation, or at least seriously impedes an assessment of affinity, and the potential for trust. Multicultural societies tend to produce pluralism in health beliefs and healthcare provision, in formal and informal sectors. So, in addition to recognised and legally sanctioned practitioners, there exists a spectrum of healing modalities provided by complementary and alternative practitioners, some of whom are genuinely well intentioned, others much less so. Who one trusts is often a matter of what one believes.

Religious beliefs are key aspects of community and personal identity which can be threatened by secularising forces, none more so than in migrant communities in which religious identity is adhered to, often tenaciously. For many, religious rituals and narratives produce a source of identity maintenance. Again, trust is directed by distinctive culture-based ontologies about the origins of suffering and relief, leading individuals within communities to conflicting beliefs about whom to trust or mistrust in help-seeking. Secular healthcare systems, or at least healthcare systems in which religion has minimal or no consideration, may not attract much trust among certain minority ethnic communities. While there are potentially negative mental health outcomes associated with service avoidance and disengagement arising from religious-cultural belief systems, it would be unwise to attribute the poor mental health of some ethnic communities to such beliefs. If ethnicity is one classification of shared identity, social class is another, additionally producing impediments to shared norms, beliefs, and values. Commonly, ethnicity and social class intersect and are mutually reinforcing.

DOI: 10.4324/9781003326687-8

The social determinants of mental illness have been identified in life-course studies for over the past two decades – poverty, bad housing, unemployment, all take their toll on health, and all more prevalent among some minority ethnic populations. It is possible that trust or mistrust in mental health services and clinicians is already conditioned by history, previous encounters, and experiences with other social institutions, and the shared community beliefs that suggest that the individual may not be treated fairly. In this chapter, we explore the concepts of trust and social capital and how these intersect with the challenges faced by minority ethnic communities, and their impact on mental health and wellbeing. While trust between individuals of different ethnic origins is obviously possible, institutional mistrust appears cemented into most of our social structures, and particularly so in mental health care.

Much of the current literature on trust is focussed on its role within social capital in determining health and wellbeing, largely in relation to a notion of a generalised trust as the basis on which people in a community are generally secure and comfortable with their fellow human beings. However, as discussed previously, this tends to simplify or ignore much of the complexity of trust – its fluidity, contextuality, and contingency. While trust and mistrust are often regarded as dimensions of individual personality, as social constructs they are varied in their determination and expression, shaped by intersectional dimensions of history, religion, political philosophy, and culture. To these national factors, may be added groups or communal factors – such as the degree of equality or disparities in a society, the distribution and access of groups to power and justice. I suggest that the problematic relationship between black and minority ethnic groups and psychiatry, is often determined by childhood circumstances and more far-reaching, the consequence of colonialism and racism; in Bourdieu's concept of habitus, 'structuring structures' predisposing the beliefs and actions of individual and communities. The academic psychiatrist and anthropologist Arthur Kleinman made the point that we often do not know 'what is at stake' for this or that patient – for example, the risks (perceived and actual) of the adolescent and the elder when faced with choices and decisions in help-seeking for mental health treatment. Moreover, the patient's identification of risk posed by either the illness or the potential contact with services cannot be uncoupled from their community's historical experiences of structural violence and other injustices.

A stranger in a strange land

There has always been some form of human migration produced by catastrophic events, natural and man-made, slavery, war, famine, colonialism, and so on. Throughout the past century or more, people migrated for economic reasons as part of an outworking of colonialism, creating sizeable diasporic migrant communities in the former empire nations. These migrations tended to be controlled and managed in ways that were aligned with the economic needs of Western states. In recent years, migration is characterised by unregulated global shifts of people due to conflict and climate change. In other words, millions of people have left their home countries or have been displaced internally because they can no longer live in these places. Many thousands have died in the attempt to settle elsewhere. The policy response of most Western states is generally hostile. In the United States, in recent years have seen the use of detention centres and the forceful separation of children from families. In Australia too, harsh policy initiatives have produced detention in off-shore islands and camps, denial of permanent residency applications and removal of free legal assistance. In Europe, there are ongoing political arguments about genuine refugees versus so-called 'economic migrants', largely creating a hostile environment for asylum-seekers but also adding to an increasingly xenophobic environment for all migrant communities (Ruhnke et al., 2024).

There are consequences for societal institutions and the individuals arising from both types of migration, those who arrived as part of a 'programme' and those who arrived as refugees and asylum seekers. First, in numerous studies across different global settings, having the status of a migrant or refugee is associated with worse mental health across a wide spectrum of disorders, than people from host or majority population. Poor mental health among refugees and migrants can be traced to the pre-migration events and circumstances, factors related to the migration journey, or the settlement experience (Bhugra & Jones, 2001). Every stage in the migration trajectory is suffused with vulnerability.

Poverty and racism

Institutionalised racism is defined as having differential levels of access, based on ethnic group, to societal goods, services, and opportunities (Williams, 1999); as such it limits access to educational attainment, employment opportunities, and social mobility. The central dimension of institutionalised racism is one of differential outcomes for different ethnic groups. However, it should be noted that such outcomes are commonly produced and/or amplified by complex social processes across multiple institutions, rather than through just one institution. Thus, institutionalised racism and its intersection with poverty, has quite defined negative impacts on access to health care, through various indirect and often opaque pathways. To describe these pathways bluntly, children from disadvantaged (poor) backgrounds are many times more likely to experience adverse childhood events (ACEs) such as sexual and violent abuse, parent mental illness and death, family break-up, and substance misuse (Gilbert et al., 2009). ACEs, in turn, will impact the individual's academic chances, again through biological, psychological, and social factors that diminish educational opportunities, access and the ability to benefit. As we explore later, these early childhood factors are associated with institutional trust, and the individual's health behaviours, help-seeking, and engagement with services. Thus, growing up with disadvantage and/or childhood trauma increases the risk of substance misuse, poor mental health and self-harm, among other things, but also reduces willingness and ability to seek professional advice or help.

Colonial legacies of mistrust

Colonialism, the subjugation, and exploitation of one population by another, and the subsequent history of mass transportation and migration of the colonised populations into alien societies has left a profound and enduring legacy down through many generations. The racist ideologies of cultural supremacy that underpinned the brutal domination of others have endured too and continue to be exploited for political ends in liberal democracies. The twin processes and effects of intergenerational trauma and racist behaviour continue to impact on the mental health of migrant and minority ethnic communities, globally. Thus, the evidence collected over almost 50 years reveals a consistent and depressing picture of high rates of alcoholism, suicide and self-harm, and mental illness among these populations compared to the majority populations. Importantly, this should not be regarded solely as a 'colour' issue; white minority groups such as the Irish in Britain have fared rather badly in terms of mental illness through several generations (Harding & Balarajan, 2001), again possibly a legacy of colonialism but also produced by racism and economic disadvantage (Leavey et al., 2007; Ryan et al., 2006). Indigenous people such as those living in North America and Australia have similarly high rates of mental illness, compared to the majority populations (Gone & Trimble, 2012). Moreover, even if we accept group differences in pathology, what accounts for this? Race as a biological explanatory concept has, quite rightly, been long dismissed, suggesting the likelihood of social environmental stressors that create an excess of mental illness among come minority communities. Indeed, a growing body of evidence points to the destructive impacts of structural inequities and discrimination that compromise physical and mental health in minority populations (Goosby et al., 2018).

Each society produces its own disadvantaged communities and disparities related to health service access and outcomes. In the United States, for example, high rates of mental health problems are found among black and Hispanic youth who also disproportionately fail to seek or receive treatment (Merikangas et al., 2011; Planey et al., 2019). Moreover, considerable ethnic disparities in psychiatric hospitalisation indicating that blacks and Native Americans are much more likely than whites to be hospitalised with blacks at greater risk of admission for schizophrenia than whites and likely to be underdiagnosed with an affective disorder. The evidence drawn from national data also suggests that Asian Americans and Pacific Islanders may be less likely than whites to be hospitalised but are committed for longer when they are, within state and county mental hospitals (Snowden & Cheung, 1990). The evidence points to blatant ethnic disparities, but whether they indicate different levels of pathology or differential access to disparate types of provision (and different quality of care) is not well understood or used misleadingly. For example, such differences may be explained by socio-economic circumstances that underpin so many risk factors for psychopathology and may require major structural changes and preventative interventions. Therefore, the higher rates of mental illness point to the problems that people have, rather than such people are problematic.

Similarly related to social inequity, some groups are disproportionately represented within the criminal justice system despite their obvious mental health needs, pointing to discrimination and injustice in the system. More widely, explanations for such differences may arise from the heightened stigma of mental illness felt within some communities and their capacity, or more likely, the resources available to families and communities for tolerance and social support. Additionally, the range of alternative mental health service provision is likely to be important. The social and cultural capital available to young middle-class white people opens a more capacious tool-kit of options when mental health is threatened, including recognition of the symptoms, knowledge of services and the ability to obtain private consultation and treatment.

In the United Kingdom, the issue of high rates of schizophrenia among the African-Caribbean community has dominated much of the academic discourse and research activity related to ethic mental illness. While these rates are contested by some within academic psychiatry as yet another indicator of Western ethnocentric ideology pathologising black people, inadvertently through misdiagnosis (Littlewood & Lipsedge, 1989) or otherwise (Fernando, 1991), it widely accepted that African-Caribbeans were entering the psychiatric system in disproportionate numbers (Bhugra et al., 1997; Kirkbride et al., 2012) and with outcomes negatively dissimilar to their white counterparts. For example, patients from this community experienced very different pathways into care; they were much more likely to be brought involuntarily into mental health units via the police (Cole et al., 1995). Compared to white British patients, minority ethnic patients were more likely to be given higher levels of anti-psychotic medication and emergency treatment (Goater et al., 1999) but less likely to offered 'talking therapies'. While patients with severe mental illness die younger than the general population irrespective of ethnicity (Das-Munshi et al., 2017), the deaths of young black men in England involuntarily detained under a section of The Mental Health Act has been a distressing and contentious subject for many years (Angiolini, 2017).

Importantly, it is a concern more generally that many of the deaths in police custody in the United Kingdom and elsewhere are of people with mental health problems, suggesting that much of the mental health supports in the community are absent or inappropriate. Nevertheless, what is commonly assumed by many within the black communities, and some within the mental health system itself is a racial bias within psychiatry; that the institution is inherently and profoundly prejudiced, and this explains why the black community in Britain mistrust the psychiatric profession and why a large proportion of young black people with mental illness disengage from care and treatment. That argument can only take us so far. The headline claims emerging from most of the academic literature on ethnicity, mental illness, and psychiatric services conceal rather than illuminate the complexity of the historical and current contexts, processes, and social dynamics that operate beneath the prevalence figures and the outcomes. Much of these social dynamics are permeated by a deep-seated mistrust originating within colonialism and still running through the migrant and minority communities. Thus, I suggest that problems of mistrust among minority ethnic and minority patients and families is not an outcome of contact within racially prejudiced clinical services, although that might also be true, but rather is a disposition determined and shaped elsewhere. There is no convincing argument that psychiatry as an institution has an interest in the arrest and incarceration of young black people within the mental health system. While the conflicts between services and communities are sometimes attributed to cultural misunderstanding, this is only one component of wider group differences and complex social arrangements that weaken or prevent the formation of trust. Importantly, the dynamics of difference and power are central.

The black community in Britain

Although there has been a black presence in Britain dating back to the Romans, the first wave of mass migration from the former colonial islands of the Caribbean arrived after 1945, strongly encouraged by the post-war government as a key element of a national rebuilding programme. In doing so, the British government tapped into a pervasive sentiment among many Windrush Caribbeans that regarded England as the 'mother country' – a mother that would look after them. As Nobrega describes, this sense of belonging and loyalty was powerfully seductive to people living in an economy with few opportunities (Nobrega, 2019, pp. 32–35).

> We came because we were coming to the mother country. Years of colonisation had indoctrinated us with a sense of belonging to England, loyalty to the Queen and country, a willingness to fight to defend this mother country and all the values of his mighty seat of empire. We learned of it in church and from our school system, our textbooks. Even our exercise books, which we handled daily in our classrooms, had the face of the beautiful Queen Elizabeth on the cover. We were not royalists and yet the Queen was wonderful (I love the Queen even now) and so we sang the national anthem. For us, the Queen was everything that was wonderful about England and about empire.

Any expectations of welcome and opportunity were soon dashed as the new migrants were greeted with hostility and discrimination in every social sphere – housing, employment, policing and the criminal justice system, education; even the established churches offered little comfort. By the 1980s the children and grandchildren of the original Windrush[2] generation were no longer prepared to endure the all-pervasive racism that manifested in unemployment, racial violence and, increasingly noticeable, high rates of psychoses and detention within psychiatric units, and especially secure forensic facilities (Coid et al., 2000). While the oppressive dimensions of psychiatry in the United Kingdom and other western states against individuals considered politically dissident, or even just socially difficult, had been stated before, this was more of a collective accusation of oppression against entire communities, and may be understood better by an examination of psychiatry's relationship with colonialism, and the need for epistemic justice by challenging 'the ways in which power, knowledge, and truth are intertwined, and highlight the manner in which discourses such as psychiatry and psychology incorporate a particular way of responding to human suffering' (Bracken et al., 2021).

Psychiatry's role in colonialism emerges most obviously in the popularly accepted scientific racism in the 19th century (Littlewood & Lipsedge, 1989).[3] While much is made of various ludicrous and self-serving racist theories made popular in 19th century, do not constitute orthodox psychiatric thinking.[4] The significance of psychiatry in its relationship to minority ethnic groups lies in its Western origins, laden with its own cultural lens and the baggage of meanings, values and priorities that had little significance to the communities and peoples dominated by western scientific ideology. Within these relationships white colonial knowledge and cultural superiority are regarded as self-evidently true and progressively such beliefs are internalised to the oppressor and the oppressed. In his book Black Skins, White Masks (1952) the psychiatrist, and political intellectual, Franz Fanon provided psychoanalytic perspectives on the internalisation of white superiority by the colonised black person and its crippling effects in the search for strategies by which to navigate living in a white-dominated world.[5] In some respects, the long-term psychological impacts of colonialism on black people (and white people) are the focus Fanon's thesis, the continuing relationship between the oppressor and the oppressed, and the struggle to exert an authentic self by migrants and the descendants of migrants are unpicked. Thus, 'what does it take to be accepted'? How should I present myself? In Fanon's schema, the paradoxical nature of these questions indicate that the struggle for acceptance and self, possesses an undermining self-consciousness that acceptance can never be achieved while sought on the other's terms. For many migrant and minority individuals, psychological destabilisation exists on a spectrum from self-doubt to self-hate. Perhaps the most obvious manifestation of self-doubt is found in the prosperous market for skin-whitening products targeted at people with black pigmentation with detrimental impacts on various levels of health (Pollock et al., 2021). Consumers using these products claim that lighter skin makes them attractive and will improve their life chances (Yusuf et al., 2019). Again, it should be stressed that this is not essentially a racial or colour issue per se but rather one of power relations irrespective of historical origins.[6]

Ethnicity and community trust

Are some ethnic communities more trusting than others? That is the basic question posed by economists Alesina and La Ferrara (2002) using data from the General Social Survey (GSS) for the United States (1974–1994) which asked respondents the question to assess *generalised trust,* that is, if they think that 'most people can be trusted'. Embedded in this study is the potential for ethnic heterogeneity in a neighbourhood to erode trust, based on the wisdom that people have less trust in those who are appear different from themselves, relative to those who appear to be similar, based on the likelihood of shared norms that assist in trust-formation. Thus, social trust is likely to be lower in ethnically diverse settings (Dinesen et al., 2020). Additionally, the potential for trust erosion in ethnically diverse settings may be explained by conflict theory and competition for material and symbolic resources (Blalock, 1967).

Although primarily interested in understanding determinants of low trust for business and economic-related purposes, their study nevertheless considered useful insights that make sense in relation to ethnic disparities in mental health. The authors noted that the factors associated with low trust are noticeable both at the level of the individual and the community characteristics. The clearest factors include a recent history of traumatic experience. The impact of traumatic events has been described as disruptive to or rupturing assumptive worlds – a 'taken for granted' sense of security that permits the flow of everyday activities. The study also revealed much lower trust among members of disadvantaged communities those who reported a history of discrimination. Strikingly too, low trust was more prevalent among people living in a racially mixed community and/or one with considerable level of income disparity. People who disliked inter-racial contacts were less trusting and more likely to live in more heterogeneous communities (Alesina & La Ferrara, 2000). As per previous studies on social capital, a positive correlation was noted between trust and participation in social activities but while blacks participated more in social and political activities, they were much less trusting than whites, even after controlling for the usual confounders. It may be that heterogeneity and low trust relate to competition among similarly disadvantaged groups for scarce resources, factionalised for political reasons. In this sense, people in more affluent communities can 'afford' to present as more tolerant and trusting because they have less contact with other groups and are not reliant on public goods and services.

Alesina and colleagues (1999) suggest that public policies have less traction in more heterogeneous areas because the member communities experience more problems in raising finance and sharing public goods largely due to mutual wariness. A seemingly banal hypothesis, it nevertheless carries a lot of weight and hides the challenges and inefficiencies within multitude of actions and transactions that are necessary in the development of interventions and services for those most in need. Thus, while culturally sensitive and informed services are vital, culturally separate services incur additional capital and other costs through reduced economies of scale. Within an environment of mistrust, costs pile up through a multiplication of legislation, checks and continuous monitoring that require additional resources to those where the parties are mutually trusting. Ultimately, contact theory which posits that prejudices and hostility decreases through contact between groups, suggests that separate services may only serve to reinforce and heighten and pre-existing intolerance and mistrust (Allport, 1979; Pettigrew & Tropp, 2005). Conversely, the growth of exchange between communities may increase trust-building. Co-operation between groups is generally a good thing, rewarding all players, unless of course intergroup cooperation is developed with aim of securing a cartel that excludes other parties. Nevertheless, the capacity of historically disadvantaged minority communities to accept that a majority community is acting in good faith without prejudice, may be limited because they have relatively more to lose.

In the United States and the United Kingdom, members of black and minority ethnic communities experience discrimination across a range of sectors such as housing, employment, education, and the criminal justice system (Kelley et al., 2017; Wood et al., 2009). It is worth stressing that while discrimination is experienced by individuals, it is also 'felt' by communities, that is, although some individuals within communities may not directly experience discrimination, they can still recognise its existence and be alert to the potential for future personal experience. In this sense perhaps, the concept of generalised trust (Rotter, 1980) may have some relevance. However, as noted previously there are considerable problems with its conceptualisation and measurement.

In most societies, the public's trust in the police is crucial to cooperation with the criminal justice system and for general neighbourhood safety. For many of the residents living in the overcrowded and disadvantaged neighbourhoods of the United States, United Kingdom, and Europe, distrust and animosity towards the police are profound and long-standing to the extent that there is a mutual regard of enmity between the police and residents (Alang et al., 2017). Again, context matters. In the United States, fear of the police is found not just among poor black residents but regarded as crucially important for survival in almost all black families regardless of social class, wealth, and neighbourhood. Prior to the origins of Black Lives Matter campaign, police victimisation and violence against young black men was a matter of concern within the black community. Black males may constitute 13% of the US population but accounted for one-quarter of police killings in 2018 and had a three-fold risk of death compared to their white counterparts (Edwards et al., 2018, 2019). Although representing only 17% of the total youth population, 62% of youths prosecuted in the adult criminal justice system are black, and have a nine-fold risk compared to white youths to receive an adult prison sentence (Arya & Augarten, 2008).

In an interesting qualitative study of neighbourhood policing, residents, and police stakeholders from North Minnesota, near St Paul, the site of some high-profile police deaths, sought to understand the deaths of young black men by police(Calvert et al., 2020). Researchers noted a dynamic cycle of vulnerability, distrust, resistance, anger, and police response to anger. Thus, defiant and disobedient behaviour was regarded as a response to 'events experienced by one's family and community; youth may have seen or heard of a family member or friend who was harmed by police, watched their father being arrested'. A culture of disobedience to law enforcement is then formed among local youths, absorbed into a generalised community members' distrust and fear of police; the defiant and aggressive behaviour of youth, the 'accumulated negative experiences' of the neighbourhood and over-policing were all seen as both and consequence of this dynamic. Into this mix, there are the familiar ingredients of poverty and high youth unemployment and the resentment that accompanies it, and the vacuum often filled by the cliché of youth 'gangs' hanging out on street corners. Ultimately, the community response of mistrust towards police emerges from fear and suspicion. This is compounded by an acknowledgement by all parties that the police fear the young black residents and undoubtedly over-react to perceived threats. Undoubtedly, racial stereotyping plays a major role in the generation of police fear. The researchers reported that participants said that most of the police they encountered 'were not from the area, did not look like them, and did not attempt to genuinely relate to community members'. Richardson and colleagues (2013) adopt the theoretical lens used by Anderson's ethnographic study, Code of the Street (Anderson, 2000), to examine how black 'street youth' in Philadelphia to make sense of, and negotiate, the lived experience of inequality, racism, and violence. Central to Anderson's thesis is the notion of respect and the imperative to use violence to gain and maintain respect – being treated right with due deference. No minor thing, making sure that one is publicly respected is a matter of life and death.

Ethnic density and mental health

As noted previously, people from migrant and minority ethnic communities are at greater risk of mental health problems than their majority counterparts and yet, in their country of origin the prevalence of these disorders appear to be like those found elsewhere. Again, the methodological rigour of studies reporting high rates of psychotic disorders provides reassurance that the disparities are unlikely to emerge through misdiagnosis.

Over the past couple of decades, a growing body of evidence has supported the possibility that the health outcomes of people from minority backgrounds may be better when they are resident in areas where their community is relatively large, compared to minority group individuals living in majority-populated areas. Often described as a group or ethnic density effect, it is sometimes analogous to a dose-response effect – the more one is surrounded by people of similar characteristics, the more 'protected' one is. Moreover, the primary or defining characteristic of minority individuals is not restricted to ethnicity as similar observations have been noted for sexuality and religion. In a recent systematic review and meta-analysis (Baker et al., 2021) found an overall 10% decrease in own-group density was associated with a 20% increase in risk for psychosis, somewhat attenuated by more finely grained analysis of ethnic minority group classifications – that is, the experience of different minority groups will vary and this may mask a wide variation in risk. This was also true of similar ethnic populations living in different national contexts – for example, Caribbeans living in the United Kingdom and those in the Netherlands. Some explanations for the group density effect, especially for more 'visible' black populations, point to the increased risk of discrimination from police and healthcare services – with consequent challenges to trust, leading to help-seeking avoidance and more coercive pathways into care (Bécares & Das-Munshi, 2013). However, while these explanations may be germane to differential post-diagnosis challenges, they fail to explain why being black in a white dominated world produces psychosis. Economic deprivation is always an obvious mechanism, but is unlikely to play a role here, simply because higher-density minority areas also tend to be the most deprived.

Ethnicity, familiarity, and mental illness

In a study using nationally representative data from Germany (Grabo & Leavey, 2023), we examined the mental health impacts associated with the perceived discrimination among refugees and asylum seekers who arrived between 2013 and 2016. There was some evidence that hostility to refugees was more virulent in the eastern region of Germany (Entorf & Lange, 2019) and thus, we hypothesised that the area of settlement (East/West) affected the prevalence of perceived discrimination of refugees and if this was related to mental health. While predictable perhaps, those who reported experience of discrimination had the worst mental health, this was significantly greater in the eastern part of Germany. Better German language proficiency was associated with a lower risk of psychological distress, indicating perhaps better integration and economic opportunities. To some extent, these differences can be explained by differing socio-structural factors between eastern and western Germany – that is, the eastern regions previously within the Soviet Union bloc, are poorer, creating greater hostility against new arrivals. We also noted that the impact of living in eastern Germany increased the risk for psychological distress among female refugees only. What seems likely is that it was their 'visibility' – not just as refugees but as Muslims from the Middle East, where headscarves are worn for religious and cultural reasons leaving them more vulnerable to racist behaviour within Germany.

Here again, factors associated with familiarity and inequality may be distinctive explanatory features of the response by the host populations and the experiences of refugees.

Historically, the eastern Germany population was much less exposed to 'foreigners' than their western counterparts, and certainly less familiar with refugees and migrant communities. In this they weren't alone, neighbouring former Soviet bloc countries such as Hungary, Poland, and the Czech Republic, all relatively more hostile to refugees, and the European Union's 'open-door' policies and strongly articulated in the political system. The anti-migrant hostility in eastern Germany may be about scarce resources but may also be explained by Allport's contact theory (Allport, 1954; Tip et al., 2019), whereby under certain circumstances, stereotyping, prejudice, and discrimination are lessened by more interpersonal contact between groups. Most people growing up in Soviet East Germany, prior to unification, were unable to watch Western television, travel abroad, or access radio broadcasts, all of which severely restricted multicultural exposure. Moreover, foreigners in Soviet East Germany, from Cuba and African countries, tended to be visitors rather than settlers, unlike the Turkish in West Germany. Until recently, ethnicity as a factor received little attention within German healthcare research and little is known about the healthcare outcomes of people from refugee and migrant backgrounds.

Social capital and mistrust

Social capital type explanations may be more plausible whereby access to consistent material and psychological resources, potentially more available within a high own-group area is protective against other adversities, and conversely, less available in low-density areas. However, as we know, social capital of the bonding kind, may not always work to everyone's advantage; while tightly bound and boundaried communities can confer benefits of trust, reciprocity, and support, such communities can also be exclusionary, denying entry, and generosity to 'outsiders', and to community members regarded as deviant in some way. Thus, what are the social and psychological experiences of non-believers in a community characterised by strong religiosity; or LGBT+ individuals in highly traditional communities where anything other than heterosexuality is considered a perversion? Individuals whose sexual identity or values and beliefs separate them from such communities are unlikely to thrive within what is often a visceral hostility. There are testimonies of many individuals who try to walk a tightrope in remaining, either in secrecy or through a punishing and usually futile demand for acceptance from the community, both at considerable mental costs (Meyer, 1995; Wolf & Platt, 2022).

Integration and trust

Regarding community, identity, and trust more generally, Berry hypothesised that migrants who fared best psychologically in host communities were those who *integrated,* a balanced position in which the migrant identifies and is involved in his or her own culture and that of the host society. *Assimilation* occurs when the migrant identifies solely with the new culture; while *Separation* is a position where the migrant is involved in the traditional culture only; and *marginalisation* is characterised by lack of involvement and rejection of both cultures. Berry argued mental health tends to vary across these four modes of settlement due to the different levels of acculturative stress that each produce. Integration has the lowest level of acculturative stress, followed by assimilation, separation, and marginalisation. While there is some evidence to confirm Berry's hypothesis on the psychological benefits of integration, it is also fair to say that it assumes that migrants are fully agentic in the matter, that there is a conscious choice in which position to adopt, when rather, often there are structural impediments (e.g., social class, finance, education, language attainment) to integration, not to mention the willingness of the host community to offer acceptance. Integration implies more than a mutual trust between the host community or at least sections of it, and the migrant, that is they sufficiently share views, beliefs, and tastes that permit integration which in multicultural societies, tend to be those of the host. Thus, aspects of the migrant's culture are relinquished or quietly faded over time, potentially permitting, but not guaranteeing, some level of trust and acceptance by the host community. However, this may come at considerable cost to the migrant.

Abdelmalek Sayad, an Algerian sociologist, and colleague of Bourdieu, provides a powerful analysis of the experiences of Muslim immigrants in France, that resonates with the contemporary social antagonisms of marginalised ethnic communities. At the heart of this is the internalisation of the racist gaze upon the migrant as being 'morally suspect' in which 'French society regards as the deviant behaviour of Muslim immigrants; wearing veils to school, statutory discrimination against women, the political use of religion, which is referred to as fundamentalism, and so on'. Sayad goes on to say that 'being conscious of the suspicion that weighs upon him' and which permeates every aspect of his life, the immigrant feels obliged to constantly anticipate it and assuage it by 'repeatedly demonstrating his good faith and his good will' (Sayad, 2004, pp. 286–287). In this, the migrant's attempts at assimilation, in Sayad's terms 'strategies of simulation and dissimulation' involve considerable efforts on self-presentation focussed on appearance and 'forms of external behaviour that are most loaded with symbolic attributes or meanings'. These efforts towards achieving the benefits associated with the dominant identity are forlorn. On one hand, the migrant will not be accepted by the dominant group but will be perceived as a traitor to his identity by his own community.

When primary aspects of culture such as dress and/or religion are not able to be negotiated, these tend to become areas of conflict within modern secular societies. In the United Kingdom and France, for example, Muslim communities have increasingly felt under pressure from state and secular forces, combined with a virulent anti-Muslim racism. The historical development of this conflict is beyond the scope of this book, but it is at least worth noting the existence of complex, relations between Islam and the West, including the colonial and political intrusion in the Muslim world by Western states, leading to the sequelae of violence and reaction from 9/11 onwards. These events and how they are manipulated by different political forces tend to generate an ecology of mutual distrust which may penetrate various social institutions in varying degrees over time. However, within Muslim, or other communities formed by a strong religious identity, there are systems of beliefs that persist without reference to external events, and these can have a considerable impact on the engagement of these communities with psychiatry, and/or medical system generally.

What's at stake – beliefs and trust

At times, beliefs and values can influence the decision-making processes involved in seeking help, such as when, and from whom, or even if one should seek help at all. Arthur Kleinman, a psychiatrist, and medical anthropologist, refers to the explanatory models of illness, a system of beliefs pertaining to a misfortune or a health problem. Psychiatry in Western societies will have a particular understanding of mental disorders, their symptoms, aetiology, and treatment, that conform to an accepted universal classificatory system such as ICD or the DSM. Nevertheless, even here, an interpretive element in the medical encounter is generally evident. Cultural psychiatry provides a framework for a meaning-centred medicine which acknowledges that illness realities are essentially semantic, and that clinical encounters and transactions allow for ambiguity of meaning. Patients and doctors may assign differential significance to the patient's experience, emphasising radically different elements of the narrative. When the patient and doctor's explanatory beliefs are consonant, there is less chance of conflict and greater likelihood of patient engagement, trust, and compliance. If dissonant, patients and their families will seek help from alternative agencies whose definition of the problem and its treatment is aligned with their beliefs and values. In this, trust, and confidence as separate but sometimes overlapping concepts are interlinked. For such individuals there is the confidence that the treating agent understands the nature of the problem but also that they can be trusted because they do not oppose the beliefs and values of the help-seeker. As part of a research programme on first episode of psychosis in ethnic groups, we examined patient and family help-seeking, and their pathways into psychiatric care (Cole et al., 1995; King et al., 1994). Many of those later diagnosed with a psychotic illness, consulted a religious or spiritual leader before contact with a psychiatrist. They did so because they and/or their families framed their symptoms as supernatural rather than medical. Most believed that they were the victims of 'black magic', witchcraft or had been possessed by demonic forces. Most, but not all, were from minority ethnic communities and these included Muslims who believed themselves to be attacked by Jinn, regarded as beings that exist outside but intruding into the human world, often causing physical and mental harm. Although the ontological reality of Jinn is not disputed within Islam, many Islamic scholars are dubious about the ubiquitous attribution of psychological problems in Muslim communities to Jinn by faith healers who make money in providing 'treatment'. Nevertheless, religious leaders in Muslim and other faith communities are wary about referring individuals with 'unusual' or worrying psychological symptoms into psychiatric services, predominantly because they regard psychiatry as secular, distrusting what they perceive as a long-standing institutionalised hostility towards religion and the pathologisation of religious beliefs and practices.

Alternative sources of power and trust

If trust is partly conditioned by belief, Freud's assessment of religion as a kind of infantilising fantasy has had an enduring effect on the relationship between religiously oriented communities and psychiatry. While few psychiatrists would declare an open hostility to religion, or religious leaders to psychiatry, the relationship has been characterised as mistrustful neighbours peering over the fence at each other. While both are in the business of dealing with human distress and misery, the level of cooperation between them is limited to say the least. The 'religiosity gap' within psychiatry, a probable consequence of its high prevalence of atheists (Bergin, 1980; Neeleman & King, 1993), provides fertile ground for anxiety and mistrust within religious and minority ethnic communities and this is a major barrier to engagement and appropriate treatment among many minority ethnic or religion-based communities. Research among religious leaders in North London, highlighted the clash between belief systems and dilemmas of the religious who have existential fears about the erosion and disappearance of religion in a secularising world (Leavey et al., 2007). For example, rabbis from the Jewish Haredi Lubavitch are reluctant to refer members of the community to psychiatric services, where they anticipate contamination by non-religious clinicians whom they perceived to be disrespectful to religious beliefs and values.

I also noted that other faith community leaders such as those in the Black Pentecostal churches are also suspicious of psychiatry but dismiss mental health services as an irrelevance, believing that human suffering is largely a problem of supernatural origin, including spirit possession which is misunderstood and misdiagnosed as a mental disorder. Emerging from downtown Los Angeles, Pentecostalism has grown exponentially and globally (Leavey, 2004; Martin, 2002), attracting adherents by its blend of spiritual and social salvation in marginalised communities. Thus, in its social and spiritual messaging, social activism and personal reform Pentecostalism provides a powerful counter-anomic approach to salvation (Martin, 2002). In doing so, Pentecostal churches often provide a public health and other programmes, such as drug rehabilitation, youth offender initiatives. These run alongside, more spiritual aspects of 'cure' through prayer, ritual healing, and deliverance from possession, intrinsic aspects of Pentecostal religious life (van Dijk, 2002). Because sickness is believed to be caused by spiritual forces, religious faith provides the cure and although this kind of explanatory model is most vigorously championed by Pentecostal clergy most of the other religious leaders I interviewed felt that mental illness was 'symptomatic of wider social and moral problems' (Leavey et al., 2016) underpinning the moral dimensions of illness experience within specific local contexts.

Encounters with spiritual leaders *or* psychiatrists have a moral dimension because of what may be at stake whereby as Kleinman argues people have 'important things to lose, to gain and to preserve' (Kleinman, 1988, p. 5) – the variation and intensity of 'things that matter' to different people across and within local worlds. In faith-based communities that are based on rigid conformity and where employment and marriage are contingent on community scrutiny that an individual (and his or her family) is free from exposure or risk to attributes or behaviours that suggest immorality, sinfulness, or mental illness. In such communities, hypervigilance and mistrust may be crucial to personal destiny and fortune.

Notes

1 Greater genetic variation exists *within* racial groups than *between* them. In fact, variation in gene frequency is 85% within racial groups, and only 15%, approximately, between the so-called racial groups. Race is now widely understood as a social construct based on phenotypic genetic expression rather than as a biological construct.
2 The Windrush was the name of the ship that brought many of the 1950s migrants to Britain.
3 While it is possible to note the historical traces it may be unfair to regard this as a direct and unbroken linkage, rather in the same way that we might see the antecedents of

modern medicine in bloodletting and its relationship with grave robbing. Thus, in fairness, psychiatry had not yet been fully established as a discipline and the psychoanalysis of Freud and Jung was still in its infancy, and generally unpopular in the mainstream.

4 Concepts such as *drapetomania*, a mental disorder proposed by the physician Samuel Cartwright for slaves who somehow irrationally felt compelled to escape.

5 Similar in some ways to Antonovsky's exploration of the difficulties of American Jews in creating 'an authentic self'.

6 The Irish in Britain are an interesting case in point. As England's first colony, the Irish experienced centuries of violent suppression, land appropriation and exploitation. Irish language and culture were systematically marginalised, and as with other colonised societies, a promulgated sense of Irish intellectual and cultural inferiority saturated all English policies towards Ireland and the Irish. The same scientific racism employed by the colonisers to justify exploitation of African and Asian colonies also produced the concept of 'negrescence' – a level of 'blackness' of which placed the Irish on a hierarchical scale much closer to the African than the Teutonic or Anglo-Saxon person (Leavey, 1998).

References

Alang, S., McAlpine, D., McCreedy, E., & Hardeman, R. (2017). Police brutality and Black health: Setting the agenda for public health scholars. *American Journal of Public Health*, *107*(5), 662–665. https://doi.org/10.2105/ajph.2017.303691

Alesina, A., Baqir, R., & Easterly, W. (1999). Public goods and ethnic divisions. *The Quarterly Journal of Economics*, *114*(4), 1243–1284.

Alesina, A., & La Ferrara, E. (2000). Participation in heterogeneous communities. *The Quarterly Journal of Economics*, *115*(3), 847–904.

Alesina, A., & La Ferrara, E. (2002). Who trusts others? *Journal of Public Economics*, *85*(2), 207–234. https://doi.org/10.1016/S0047-2727(01)00084-6

Allport, G. W. (1954). *The nature of prejudice*. Addison-Wesley.

Allport, G. W. (1979). *The nature of prejudice (25th anniversary ed.)*. Addison-Wesley.

Anderson, E. (2000). *Code of the street: Decency, violence, and the moral life of the inner city*. WW Norton & Company.

Angiolini, E. (2017). *Report of the independent review of deaths and serious incidents in police custody*. https://assets.publishing.service.gov.uk/government/uploads/system/uploads/attachment_data/file/655401/Report_of_Angiolini_Review_ISBN_Accessible.pdf

Arya, N., & Augarten, I. (2008). Critical condition: African-American youth in the justice system. Available at SSRN https://ssrn.com/abstract=1892957.

Baker, S. J., Jackson, M., Jongsma, H., & Saville, C. W. N. (2021). The ethnic density effect in psychosis: A systematic review and multilevel meta-analysis. *British Journal of Psychiatry*, *219*(6), 632–643. https://doi.org/10.1192/bjp.2021.96

Bécares, L., & Das-Munshi, J. (2013). Ethnic density, health care seeking behaviour and expected discrimination from health services among ethnic minority people in England. *Health & Place*, *22*, 48–55.

Bergin, A. E. (1980). Psychotherapy and religious values. *Journal of Consulting and Clinical Psychology*, *48*, 95–105.

Bhugra, D., & Jones, P. (2001). Migration and mental illness. *Advances in Psychiatric Treatment*, *7*, 216–222.

Bhugra, D., Leff, J., Mallett, R., Der, G., Corridan, B., & Rudge, S. (1997). Incidence and outcome of schizophrenia in whites, African-Caribbeans and Asians in London. *Psychological Medicine*, *27*(4), 791–798. https://doi.org/10.1017/s0033291797005369

Blalock, H. (1967). *Toward a theory of minority-group relations*. Wiley.

Bracken, P., Fernando, S., Alsaraf, S., Creed, M., Double, D., Gilberthorpe, T., Hassan, R., Jadhav, S., Jeyapaul, P., Kopua, D., Parsons, M., Rodger, J., Summerfield, D., Thomas, P., & Timimi, S. (2021). Decolonising the medical curriculum: Psychiatry faces particular challenges. *Anthropology & Medicine, 28*(4), 420–428. https://doi.org/10.1080/1364847 0.2021.1949892

Calvert, C. M., Brady, S. S., & Jones-Webb, R. (2020). Perceptions of violent encounters between police and young Black men across stakeholder groups. *Journal of Urban Health, 97*(2), 279–295. https://doi.org/10.1007/s11524-019-00417-6

Coid, J., Kahtan, N., Gault, S., & Jarman, B. (2000). Ethnic differences in admissions to secure forensic psychiatry services. *British Journal of Psychiatry, 177*, 241–247.

Cole, E., Leavey, G., King, M., Johnson-Sabine, E., & Hoar, A. (1995). Pathways to care for patients with a first episode of psychosis: A comparison of ethnic groups. *British Journal of Psychiatry, 167*, 770–776.

Das-Munshi, J., Chang, C. -K., Dutta, R., Morgan, C., Nazroo, J., Stewart, R., & Prince, M. J. (2017). Ethnicity and excess mortality in severe mental illness: A cohort study. *The Lancet Psychiatry, 4*(5), 389–399. https://doi.org/10.1016/S2215-0366(17)30097-4

Dinesen, P. T., Schaeffer, M., & Sønderskov, K. M. (2020). Ethnic diversity and social trust: A narrative and meta-analytical review. *Annual Review of Political Science, 23*, 441–465. https://doi.org/10.1146/annurev-polisci-052918-020708

Edwards, F., Esposito, M. H., & Lee, H. (2018). Risk of police-involved death by race/ethnicity and place, United States, 2012-2018. *American Journal of Public Health, 108*(9), 1241–1248. https://doi.org/10.2105/ajph.2018.304559

Edwards, F., Lee, H., & Esposito, M. (2019). Risk of being killed by police use of force in the United States by age, race-ethnicity, and sex. *Proceedings of the National Academy of Sciences of the United States of America, 116*(34), 16793–16798. https://doi.org/10.1073/pnas.1821204116

Entorf, H., & Lange, M. (2019). Refugees welcome? Understanding the regional heterogeneity of anti-foreigner hate crimes in Germany. *Understanding the Regional Heterogeneity of Anti-Foreigner Hate Crimes in Germany (January 30, 2019). ZEW-Centre for European Economic Research Discussion Paper* (19-005).

Fanon, F. (1952). *Black skin, white masks*. Grove Press.

Fernando, S. (1991). *Mental health, race and culture*. Macmillan in association with MIND.

Gilbert, R., Widom, C. S., Browne, K., Fergusson, D., Webb, E., & Janson, S. (2009). Burden and consequences of child maltreatment in high-income countries. *Lancet, 373*(9657), 68–81. https://doi.org/10.1016/s0140-6736(08)61706-7

Goater, N., King, M., Cole, E., Leavey, G., & Sabine, E. (1999). Ethnicity and outcome of psychosis. *British Journal of Psychiatry, 175*, 34–42.

Gone, J. P., & Trimble, J. E. (2012). American Indian and Alaska native mental health: Diverse perspectives on enduring disparities. *Annual Review of Clinical Psychology, 8*, 131–160. https://doi.org/10.1146/annurev-clinpsy-032511-143127

Goosby, B. J., Cheadle, J. E., & Mitchell, C. (2018). Stress-related biosocial mechanisms of discrimination and African American health inequities. *Annual Review of Sociology, 44*(1), 319–340.

Grabo, J., & Leavey, G. (2023). Geographical disparities and settlement factors and mental health of refugees living in Germany. *International Journal of Environmental Research and Public Health, 20*(5). https://doi.org/10.3390/ijerph20054409

Harding, S., & Balarajan, R. (2001). Mortality of third generation Irish people living in England and Wales: Longitudinal study. *British Medical Journal, 322*, 466–467.

Kelley, N., Khan, O., & Sharrock, S. (2017). *Racial prejudice in Britain today*. NatCen Social Research and Runnymede Trust.

King, M., Coker, E., Leavey, G., Hoar, A., & Johnstone-Sabine, E. (1994). Incidence of psychotic illness in London: Comparison of ethnic groups. *British Medical Journal, 309*, 1115–1119.

Kirkbride, J. B., Errazuriz, A., Croudace, T. J., Morgan, C., Jackson, D., Boydell, J., Murray, R. M., & Jones, P. B. (2012). Incidence of schizophrenia and other psychoses in England, 1950-2009: A systematic review and meta-analyses. *PLOS One*, *7*(3), e31660. https://doi.org/10.1371/journal.pone.0031660

Kleinman, A. (1988). *Rethinking psychiatry: From cultural category to personal experience*. Free Press.

Leavey, G. (1998). The denigration of the Irish. In Susan Grenfield (Ed.), *Hate thy neighbour: Dividing lines of race and colour - Mindfield Issue 1*. Camden Press.

Leavey, G. (2004). Identity and belief within black Pentecostalism. In D. Kelleher, & G. Leavey (Eds.), *Identity and health* (pp. 37–58). Routledge.

Leavey, G., Loewenthal, K., & King, M. (2007). Challenges to sanctuary: The clergy as a resource for mental health care in the community. *Social Science and Medicine*, *65*, 548–559.

Leavey, G., Loewenthal, K., & King, M. (2016). Locating the social origins of mental illness: The explanatory models of mental illness among clergy from different ethnic and faith backgrounds. *Journal of Religion and Health*, *55*(5), 1607–1622. https://doi.org/10.1007/s10943-016-0191-1

Leavey, G., Rozmovits, L., Ryan, L., & King, M. (2007). Explanations of depression among Irish migrants in Britain. *Social Science & Medicine*, *65*, 231–244.

Littlewood, R., & Lipsedge, M. (1989). *Aliens and alienists* (2nd ed.). Unwin Hyman.

Martin, D. (2002). *Pentecostalism: The world their parish*. Blackwell.

Merikangas, K. R., He, J.-p, Burstein, M., Swendsen, J., Avenevoli, S., Case, B., Georgiades, K., Heaton, L., Swanson, S., & Olfson, M. (2011). Service utilization for lifetime mental disorders in U.S. adolescents: Results of the National Comorbidity Survey–Adolescent Supplement (NCS-A). *Journal of the American Academy of Child & Adolescent Psychiatry*, *50*(1), 32–45. https://doi.org/10.1016/j.jaac.2010.10.006

Meyer, I. H. (1995). Minority stress and mental health in gay men. *Journal of Health and Social Behavior*, *36*(1), 38–56.

Neeleman, J., & King, M. (1993). Psychiatrists' religious attitudes in relation to the clinical practice: A survey of 231 psychiatrists. *Acta Psychiatrica Scandanavica*, *88*, 420–424.

Nobrega, B. M. (2019). 'Why did we come'. In J. Webb, R. Westmaas, M. del Pilar Kaladeen, & W. Tantam (Eds.), *Memory, migration and (De)Colonisation in the Caribbean and beyond*. University of London Press.

Pettigrew, T. F., & Tropp, L. R. (2005). Allport's intergroup contact hypothesis: Its history and influence. In J. F. Dovidio, P. Glick, & L. A. Rudman (Eds.), *On the nature of prejudice* (pp. 262–277). Blackwell. https://doi.org/10.1002/9780470773963.ch16

Planey, A. M., Smith, S. M., Moore, S., & Walker, T. D. (2019). Barriers and facilitators to mental health help-seeking among African American youth and their families: A systematic review study. *Children and Youth Services Review*, *101*, 190–200. https://doi.org/10.1016/j.childyouth.2019.04.001

Pollock, S., Taylor, S., Oyerinde, O., Nurmohamed, S., Dlova, N., Sarkar, R., Galadari, H., Manela-Azulay, M., Chung, H. S., Handog, E., & Kourosh, A. S. (2021). The dark side of skin lightening: An international collaboration and review of a public health issue affecting dermatology. *International Journal of Women's Dermatology*, *7*(2), 158–164. https://doi.org/10.1016/j.ijwd.2020.09.006

Richardson, J. B. Jr., Brown, J., & Van Brakle, M. (2013). Pathways to early violent death: The voices of serious violent youth offenders. *American Journal of Public Health*, *103*(7), e5–16. https://doi.org/10.2105/ajph.2012.301160

Rotter, J. B. (1980). Interpersonal trust, trustworthiness, and gullibility. *American Psychologist*, *35*(1), 1–7. https://doi.org/10.1037/0003-066X.35.1.1

Ruhnke, S. A., Hertner, L., Köhler, J., & Kluge, U. (2024). Social ecological determinants of the mental distress among Syrian refugees in Lebanon and Turkey: A transnational perspective. *Social Science & Medicine, 346*, 116700. https://doi.org/10.1016/j.socscimed.2024.116700

Ryan, L., Leavey, G., Golden, A., Blizard, R., & King, M. (2006). Depression in Irish Migrants to London: A case control study. *British Journal of Psychiatry, 188*, 560–566.

Sayad, A. (2004). *The suffering of the immigrant.* Polity.

Senior, P. A., & Bhopal, R. (1994). Ethnicity as a variable in epidemiological research. *BMJ, 309*(6950), 327–330. https://doi.org/10.1136/bmj.309.6950.327

Snowden, L. R., & Cheung, F. K. (1990). Use of inpatient mental health services by members of ethnic minority groups. *American Psychologist, 45*(3), 347–355. https://doi.org/10.1037//0003-066x.45.3.347

Tip, L. K., Brown, R., Morrice, L., Collyer, M., & Easterbrook, M. J. (2019). Improving refugee well-being with better language skills and more intergroup contact. *Social Psychological and Personality Science, 10*(2), 144–151.

van Dijk, R. (2002). The soul is the stranger: Ghanaian Pentecostalism and the diasporic contestation of 'flow' and 'individuality. *Culture and Religion, 3*(1), 49–65.

Williams, D. R. (1999). Race, socioeconomic status, and health. The added effects of racism and discrimination. *Annals of the New York Academy of Sciences, 896*, 173–188. https://doi.org/10.1111/j.1749-6632.1999.tb08114.x

Wolf, J. K., & Platt, L. F. (2022). Religion and sexual identities. *Current Opinion in Psychology, 48*, 101495. https://doi.org/10.1016/j.copsyc.2022.101495

Wood, M., Hales, J., Purdon, S., Sejersen, T., & Hayllar, O. (2009). *A test for racial discrimination in recruitment practice in British cities.*

Yusuf, M. A., Mahmoud, N. D., Rirash, F. R., Stoff, B. K., Liu, Y., & McMichael, J. R. (2019). Skin lightening practices, beliefs, and self-reported adverse effects among female health science students in Borama, Somaliland: A cross-sectional survey. *International Journal of Women's Dermatology, 5*(5), 349–355.

Chapter 9

Stigma and Trust

Despite the recent surge in so-called 'culture wars', engineered to contrive a divisive and hostile atmosphere around issues that matter to different social groups, policies related to the inclusion of marginalised and disadvantaged populations has managed to gain a slight foothold in many Western liberal democracies. Nevertheless, the struggle for policy acknowledgement points to structural barriers that deny or limit access to assets and activities that others may take for granted. Even the language of minority and majority populations, highlights a distinction that requires consideration about the needs, rights, and entitlement within this binary. Thus, a commonplace assumption in democratic societies suggests that if most people (the majority) believe this or that, or have similar goals and common requirements, then the few (the minority) must acquiesce.[1] The rights of minorities are sometimes, often poorly, protected by legislation, but these rights tend to be asserted, not given, following a long history of oppression and counter struggle – think of freedoms for black people, women, workers, and homosexuality. Moreover, even though the civil and human rights of various populations are enshrined in law, discriminatory behaviour, often justified as cultural norms, is highly prevalent, visible, and not easily challenged. The least visible and easiest to invalidate are least likely to assert these rights, despite an abundance of human rights legislation.

Human beings in most cultures are programmed or primed, at least, to create boundaries – distinguishing between what is considered good or bad, edible, and inedible, valued, and valueless. The concept of *homophily* describes a general human propensity to seek out other people of similar appearance or other characteristics. Connecting and being surrounded with others similar to ourselves, narcissistic as it appears, may instinctively serve to produce feelings of security and alleviate anxiety. Inside this hall of mirrors, we define ourselves by the characteristics we see around us. In doing so we also define who we are not. Depending on the context, such boundaries are often ritualised and sometimes policed. Often too, they become internalised as habits (or habitus) (Bourdieu, 1977) and have a lifespan way beyond their original purpose. The anthropologist Mary Douglas in her seminal book *Purity and Danger (2002)* points to the hygienic protection through strict dietary rules and behaviours among ancient Jewish communities living in a hot

DOI: 10.4324/9781003326687-9

and challenging climate. Douglas suggested that such restrictions may appear bizarre to the outsider but have obvious relevance for religious Jews living in secular societies as a way of reinforcing religious identity, symbolic expressions of being different to, and separate from, other religious and ethnic groups.[2] Being different matters. As discussed in this chapter on stigma, being different also has implications for intergroup and interpersonal trust.

The boundaries between risk and trust are mutually reinforcing at all levels – social, ideological, psychological, and physical. Transgression of boundaries may result in disapproving looks or banishment from the community. It is also true that boundaries have their origins in authority and power. Culture isn't a necessarily rigid set of rules but the degree to which they are adaptable and subject to change, are dependent on the source of power to enforce the rules and the boundaries. Individuals leaving for foreign shores were often regarded by their native families and communities as vulnerable to 'being lost', or rather, in danger of losing religious or cultural knowledge and habits – becoming different. Thus, valued aspects of community origins and membership appear threatened (or polluted) through contact with alien communities and their beliefs. Ethnic and religious diasporas continue to exist through the desire for identity maintenance, a direct transportation of beliefs and habits from one country to another, overcoming and obliterating other national boundaries in the process. However, while the benefits derived by some individuals and groups through a given identity and the sense of community and belonging that this offers, will ensure preservation and connection, this is not the case when an identity is assigned by others. An individual might *belong* to a tightly knit ethnic and/or religious community, in the sense that their religious or ethnic background indicates a primary identity for social administrative purposes but receives no sense of this *belonging* through other members of the community. Rejection such as this happens when the group feels threatened or at risk in some way.

Living in the exterior – mental illness and social exclusion

People living with severe and enduring mental illness, whichever country, or community they reside, are among the most socially excluded individuals in society. They are generally invisible and unthought of until occasionally, the media highlights their existence through a shocking media story of a random act of violence. Even though, people with schizophrenia are more likely to be victims of violence and that murders are more likely to be committed by a family member or an individual without a mental illness, such stories awaken the lightly dormant anxieties that accompany historical stereotypes of madness. It is said that in the medieval period, people deemed mad would be sent off on long sea voyages, in a belief that the ship's movement was curative. They may also have simply been escorted by sailors, at a price, to dump their 'cargo' of unfortunates in some distant port.

Mostly, one assumes, it was a removal, as far and for as long as possible the embarrassing or difficult family member.

> The madman's voyage is at once a rigorous division and an absolute Passage. In one sense, it simply develops, across a half-real, half-imaginary geography, the madman's *liminal* position on the horizon of medieval concern - a position made real at the same by the madman's privilege of being confined within the city gates: his exclusion must enclose him; if he cannot and must not have another prison than the threshold itself, he is kept at the point of passage. He is put in the exterior of the interior, and conversely. A highly symbolic position, which will doubtless remain his until our own day, if we are willing to admit what was formerly a visible fortress of order has now become a castle of our conscience.
>
> (Foucault, 1977, p. 11)

Foucault's (1977) work on social responses to madness in Europe over several centuries, describes an alternative reaction, that is the display of people deemed insane, noting that as late as 1815, the Bethlehem hospital ('Bedlam') 'exhibited lunatics for a penny every Sunday' (in Madness and Civilization, p. 68). In Paris and other cities, madness had become a spectacle, entertainment for the new urbanites. Foucault also observes the disappearance of leprosy from European cities during the 12th to the 14th centuries but the role of scapegoat that the leper served needed a replacement, finding it in the insane.

Until the arrival of the concept of care in the community, people deemed to have mental illness were placed in large psychiatric hospitals, commonly in distant and isolated rural locations. The asylum system in the United Kingdom and elsewhere were largely developments of the Victorian era, made possible by public coffers swollen from profits of industrialisation and reservoirs of wealth spilling over from the slave trade and colonial enterprise. Orderly management of systems and workers required the removal of the unfit far from the regular processes. In the late 20th century, the development of psychopharmacology, albeit crudely blunt and problematic offered the chance of a different kind of 'containment'. Thus, the suppression of excessive and prominent symptoms, combined with a genuine need for reform of the old psychiatric hospital system, permitted the closure of the large 'asylums' and the decanting of people with mental illness into the community. Even following the transition from large asylums to life in the community, Foucault's wry observation on the location of the mentally ill within 'the exterior of the interior, and conversely', still resonates truthfully about the community's relationship with mental illness. Thus, people with severe mental illness (SMI)[3] in the 1990s were decanted into neighbourhoods, commonly urban, poor and run-down areas, and despite the term 'care in the community' it would be difficult to describe this is as being part of a community in any credible understanding of the term – a sense of belonging, participation in community activities, and a connection with others offering mutual support – affective and material. In this way, Foucault's observation is perceptive. People with a history of severe mental illness are to be found in the midst of our cities (interior) but marginalised and excluded (exterior). The mentally ill, once termed 'aliens', may still be considered as abandoned on foreign shores with various boundaries imposed upon them by families, institutions, and clinicians. In the United Kingdom, due to the closure of many local mental health rehabilitation facilities patients are commonly treated in units often hundreds of miles from their home location (Killaspy, 2006). In poor communities which are already under severe economic pressure, deinstitutionalisation has more dramatic consequences. In 2016, the Gauteng Department of Health in South Africa ceased funding a large 2000 bed facility discharging vulnerable people with psychosocial disability into unregistered community residential facilities. Consequently, more than 140 people died (Patel et al., 2018).

'Mad, bad and dangerous to know' – the weaponising of mistrust

The sociologist Erving Goffman used the word stigma as a useful construct to consider the impact of labelling of people as having some negative characteristic or other that distinguish them from other members of the community (Goffman, 1963). Borrowed the term from the Greeks – a stigma is an indelible mark, burnt or carved into the skin (see also stigmata), and identifying the bearers as shameful and unworthy persons, criminals, or slaves for example, and thus unacceptable to a normatively decent society. More recently, stigma theory has opened the definition to include aspects of labelling and stereotyping whereby the negative identity once fixed, accrues other attributes which are almost impossible to shake off. The person thus stigmatised is then invalidated and socially excluded. Such stigmas have been used to denigrate, marginalise, and attack various individuals and communities – people with disabilities, ethnic minorities, LGBTQ+, the poor, and those with neurodevelopmental or mental health problems. While many such stigmatising attributes are not universal or fixed, and may be malleable to social and cultural change, mental illness remains obdurately potent across time and place.

Trust (and Mistrust) plays a critical role in the process of stigmatisation with considerable implications for the health and social outcomes of people who experience a severe mental illness, regardless of diagnosis. First, the stigmatising impacts of mental illness are calculated by the individual and his or her individual. What will the damage be if other people in the community know about this? What will be their response – sympathetic or hostile? Can the illness be concealed – are the symptoms noticeable by others? How long will it last and will they be able to maintain their place at work (or college)? The person with the illness (or their family) may have no prior knowledge on which to base a strategy but stigmatising attitudes to mental illness, as part of a tacit cultural knowledge, do not require explicit guidance. Like racism and misogyny, negative beliefs and attitudes are in the social ether – they don't have to be discussed or regularly expressed, but their existence is communicated, nevertheless. Within such environments, stigmatising beliefs and attitudes are taken for granted.

The existence of dehumanising beliefs tends to influence the behaviour of the victims in one of several ways, resistance, or avoidance. Anticipating the dangers, one either avoids the environment or confronts it. Thus, people living with mental health problems can, and do, anticipate the hostility and other potential disadvantages should their illness become known; however, the anticipated response will depend greatly on the diagnosis, symptoms and how these are presented. While many people live with depression or anxiety throughout their lives and may never have sought professional help, often because they remain able to function – commonly through employment or family support, other disorders create more disruption. The symptoms and functional challenges of other mental disorders such as schizophrenia and bi-polar, make the maintenance of regular activities and relationships somewhat unlikely, without recourse to professional support and treatment. The objective disruption to life and relationships propels contact with clinicians, even if the patient isn't the one to initiate it.

The calculation of risk by the patient and his or her family is sometimes determined by the level and type of information that they hold – about the seriousness of the person's mental health problems, how they will be treated by the mental health services and the personal and social impacts of people in their own community, family networks, friends, and colleagues. Moreover, stigma negatively impacts on engagement with treatment and satisfaction with services; it also associated with poor clinical and social outcomes (Corrigan et al., 2016). Among the public, there is a general poverty of mental health literacy (Jorm, 2000), as it is sometimes called, knowledge about the symptoms and course of different mental disorders, and how one should respond to these. The problem of ignorance is compounded by stigmatising attitudes not just about mental illness, but also the clinicians, services, and facilities that exist to help.

The impact of stigma

Despite the general disposition of trust towards the health profession, the bleak images of the old Victorian asylums have seeped into the collective imagination long after the closure of such places, and to such an extent that families of people with obvious mental health problems, do not trust psychiatric services to behave with kindness and compassion. In a study of suicide (Leavey et al., 2016), we reviewed the primary care records of people who died by suicide over a four-year period; we also interviewed many of their bereaved family members and general practitioners who experienced a suicide in their practice. We explored with the participants the causal attributions they held about the suicide and the help-seeking pathways, if any, that were negotiated prior to the death. These interviews reveal much about attitudes to mental illness and the stigma that prevents trust in others and the strategies used by suicidal people to avoid a diagnosis and/ or psychiatric treatment. Converting emotional and psychological problems into a somatic presentation appears to be one form of resolving the shame associated with mental illness of problems, resulting in misrecognition of underlying affective disorders (Kirmayer & Robbins, 1996; Rosendal et al., 2005). For others, the stigma attached to mental illness posed a substantial threat to reputation, position, or role; again, leading to concealment of mental health problems and/or failure to seek appropriate help. Such fears extended to close family members and spouses. In the following interview, one woman described how her sister, admitted to hospital following a suicide attempt, was fearful that her husband would leave her. Whether these fears are grounded in her illness or through a reasonable assessment of her husband's prejudice, is unclear. However, the existence of these beliefs confirms their social potency.

> She was taken to [the psychiatric hospital] that day and got her stomach pumped. She just got out of there again immediately. She said she was scared they would offer her psychiatric help because she said if they did '[my husband] *would never take me back again – if there was any way that I was ever treated for mental health problems.*' ...she said, '*I can't stay in here any longer than necessary.*'

Again, similar narratives highlight the actuality or perception of deeply stigmatising attitudes towards mental illness within the local community. In the following quote, the full weight of stigma may emerge following the voluntary admission and contact, deterring further contact:

> After a suicide attempt, he went into a [psychiatric hospital] voluntarily. I think from his point of view, hospitalisation was detrimental to his mental health because when he left there, he felt that the stigma attached to that was unbearable and given the mindset of the community that he lived in, there was such stigma attached to that ...
>
> (Brother)

> No, I'm not going over to that place ... Sure the whole of [town name] will know there's something wrong with you.
>
> (Sister)

We also noted that some people had communicated their suicidal intentions, directly or indirectly, but refused to seek professional help, to the distress of family members. The following accounts show the complexity within family dynamics and uncertainty of getting emergency help. What is clearly a dilemma for many relatives confronted by mental illness in the family, is a psychological and emotional 'stalemate' in which they are self-conscious about the potential perception of 'betrayal' of the person who is ill and alternatively, a desire to prevent his or her mental deterioration. This dilemma underscores the ambiguity of the illness, its symbolic importance, and what must be negotiated between lay and professional actors. These dynamics are seldom found in other diagnostic areas. Thus, relatives and friends of people experiencing heart attack or stroke symptoms tend not to contest the need for medical intervention, worry about the type of intervention, or where the intervention will be provided and who will know about it. Strikingly, some relatives, even when they are aware of the suicide risk, appear paralysed

> We knew that she was feeling suicidal; she had said that. But she did not want … I asked her about going to the GP and getting medical help and all that, she didn't want that, and I didn't push it.
>
> (Sister)

> So, the alarm bells were ringing. […] But at that stage, he was in line to see a psychiatrist. At the time, I was attending a counsellor, for depression, so I phoned her and asked her what I should do; could I get a doctor to sign him into [the psychiatric hospital] because I was a bit worried, and she said we'd have real problems to get a doctor to sign him in unless he goes willingly. So, we tried to persuade him to go willingly to [the hospital]. He wasn't having any of that, so it came to a stalemate.
>
> (P34, Brother)

While relatives commonly attributed some of this avoidance behaviour to the stigma associated with mental health institutions generally, in other cases, there was a concern about specific psychiatric hospitals. Northern Ireland is comprised of small, highly networked communities. This perception of proximity and transparency appears to exacerbate the degree and impact of stigma. To some degree, it is unclear in many of the narratives whether the 'fear' of psychiatric institutions is historical, that is, embedded in the folk memory of the asylum, or perhaps, determined by a more current local familiarity, but certainly there is some recognition that these may be overvalued beliefs held by entirely by the patient but in some cases, shared by their families.

> The family that I came from would be a well-known family who would know everybody around the area, and he had it in his head that because of that, everybody knew that he had been up there [the inpatient psychiatric unit], and to be honest, I have yet to hear anybody mention it. There is nobody outside of our family I've ever heard even mention it, apart from his close friends.
>
> (Brother)

Perhaps surprisingly, an opposition to psychiatric hospital admissions by families was noted, as was the case of one sister:

> But he went into [the local hospital], which I didn't agree because the things that goes on inside that hospital is not … it's not right.

In some cases, family members intervened to block a referral to hospital. In the following excerpt, we note a vehement rejection of hospitalisation in a psychiatric unit:

> She said, '*I'm going into hospital.*' '*Right,*' I said, '*That's okay.*' So, I went down and phoned my brother and said to him and he came down and in her own house and they had a fallout and he told her to get a grip of herself and pull herself together and this was stupid, her going into [name of hospital].

> (P49, Sister)

In this case, this man and his brother lacked any direct personal experience of the hospital. Similarly, although described in harsher terms, this friend does not consider the option of inpatient psychiatric treatment as viable because he would find the treatment of patients in these institutions as inhumane:

> There is nowhere for people to go with mental health problems. [The mental health hospital], as I say, when you get into [there], you wouldn't put your dog in it.

> (Friend)

Over millennia, the denigration, and occasionally the destruction, of a tribal or political leader, was successfully accomplished by deeming him or her as mad. The conferral of insanity meant that the person was 'not fit' to lead, and in extremis, not fit to live. The individual's intelligence, judgement, sincerity, compassion, and morality were all rendered as questionable. Denigration previously done within small, localised settings can now be achieved on a universal scale. Twenty-four-hour television news, omnipresent internet-based coverage, and social media, replete with clever editing and memes can render the most innocent and banal of expressions, facial or verbal, as questionable or spectacularly weird- signifying someone's insanity, latent or otherwise, and unfit for office. Although many politicians can be arrogant, narcissistic, and ignorant, their conduct does not fit within the acceptable boundaries of a contemporary psychiatric diagnosis. However, one doesn't have to hold high office or be famous to be undermined by innuendo of insanity.[4] Nevertheless, in the political sphere, we damn people with the soubriquet of madness in a way that people with a chronic illness or disability would ever be impugned. Sadly, the denigration and devaluation of individuals and groups through the weaponisation of mistrust in madness has an equally long human history – related to power and the ability and desire to dominate others.

Stigma as power

The term 'gaslighting' has its origins in a 1938 drama called Gaslight and has become popular in contemporary western culture – generally meaning a concerted process of manipulation and deceit designed to undermines another person's sense of reality, so that the individual is led on a controlled pathway to self-doubt, and eventual insanity. Although often used to describe an abusive relationship, 'gaslighting' has also been used in politics to characterise forms of harassment, often played out in the mass media, or deceiving the public for political ends through modern marketing and communication techniques. Central to gaslighting is the determination to discredit the individual (or group) as perceived by others and themselves.

Link and Phelan, leading researchers and theorists on the stigma of mental illness, have recently turned to the concept of stigma power (Link & Phelan, 2014). Based on Bourdieu's concepts of symbolic power and misrecognition, they turn the focus from the stigmatised to the stigmatiser in a consideration of who and why stigma might be value to the people who 'weaponize' it. Link and Phelan regard stigma, as having symbolic power – a cultural evaluation of things – for example, goods, arts, manners and beliefs, qualities placed within a hierarchy of 'good' or 'bad'. The question posed by Bourdieu is who can impose these judgements, or by processes do they come to be regarded as natural or having a taken for granted 'truth'. Thus, symbolic power operates within grammar or etiquette – tastes that have no intrinsic or objective values but are co-opted in distinguishing so-called high and low social classes, the 'cultured' from the 'common' and so on. Such valuations or tastes become reified into a symbolic framework through which people (and communities) are assessed as having, or lacking in, qualities or characteristics that are prized. Again, power is enacted and made visible through the ability of one social group to make such qualities to be 'obviously' superior.

Thus, the use of stigma may be of value to some sectors in that it permits a level of invisibility for discriminatory and/or behaviours in the service of outcomes that might otherwise be considered unacceptable. The processes achieve misrecognition through indirect and concealed in various taken for granted cultural circumstances. The goal of stigma power is to discreetly achieve the social exclusion of the stigmatised – to stay 'in', 'down', or 'away' as expressed by Link and Phelan. They argue that although the most obvious form of discrimination is the person-to-person type but when done blatantly may incur sanctions for the stigmatiser – such behaviour may simply reflect badly among one's peers or may provoke processes related to employment rights legislation. While it may be possible to recognise individual acts of discrimination against people with mental illness in the way that Link and Phelan suggest may result in a collective outcome which suggests structural or institutional discrimination, their position lacks a more nuanced consideration of the contexts and mechanisms through which discrimination is enacted. First, we need to consider the specific site (or in Bourdieu's terms, 'field') of discrimination. First, to speak of the stigma relating to 'mental illness' wrongly suggests a single entity when, of course, there are multiple diagnostic categories, each with their own specific outer and inner manifestations – how the symptoms are presented to others and how these make the person feel. These too are associated differentially upon the disorders' course, impacts, and outcomes. Thus, each disorder tends to be regarded differently by those that experience it, and differently responded to by the community in which they live. Each problem is assessed for its potential risk to the person, family, and community.

Culturally, there are major variations in experience and response, and these too are subject to change over time. Moral perspectives and injunctions tend to wither in more individualistic modernity. A mental health problem that was stigmatised in some Western societies ten years ago may be much less of a problem for the bearer today, permitting higher levels of help seeking in some circles. While an admission of a depression or an eating disorder, or a personal struggle with alcohol and drugs may once have put a dark question mark over most careers, it is now engagingly fashionable for celebrities and professional royalty to voice their problems in highly confessional and public forums. Such problems, however described, are now increasingly absorbed into narratives of brave survival and resilience. Rather than hidden from neighbourly curiosity, the experience of mental illnesses now fill the content of autobiographies and television chat-shows.

Again however, the contextual circumstances of the individual who experiences a mental health problem will also determine or at least influence, its course and outcome – the risk and the anticipated response. The concept of anticipated stigma shifts the focus on beliefs and behaviour from the potential stigmatisers in society to those of whom we tend to think of the stigmatised. An individual who begins to develop a depressive illness may not reveal these problems or seek help from others not because they feel shame or embarrassment, but because of what else might be at stake beyond personal dignity. The world is a relatively unforgiving place for an isolated, single-parent woman dependent on the wages from low paid and precarious employment. Depression and anxiety may be the logical consequence of such circumstances but the perceived or actual risks to her income and children, allow little room for trust. Why would someone in these circumstances expect a favourable outcome from people who, at least theoretically, might be able to help?

Undoubtedly, employers and bosses don't necessarily welcome 'people with problems' – they may not even like to employ people who have had problems many years ago, calculating a risk that such problems may return. Such employers may believe that health problems and disabilities, whatever they might be, are likely to incur costs, either through adjustments in the workplace or days lost through illness. They may distrust the individual to carry out their work efficiently or get along with other people. Much of these beliefs and attitudes arise from ignorance and prejudice and while the appointment of such people as managers in an organisation is a concern, they exist, clearly. However, many managers lack competencies in the detection of common mental health problems such as depression and anxiety in the workforce and lack awareness who may be experiencing problems, unless the employee's attendance or ability to function is highly compromised.

One definition of a psychiatric disability is based on the ability to attain age-appropriate goals due to a mental health problem that persists over time (Corrigan et al., 2008). The issues of stigma and trust related to mental illness must be considered in the context of specific disorders, their aetiology, symptoms, and sequelae. So, how might society respond to a young man who started experiencing voices and visual hallucinations in his adolescence? The evidence suggests very poorly. Regardless of the economic, political, or cultural contexts in which they are located, unemployment among people with severe mental illness is extremely high. They are also more likely to be single and/or to lack academic qualifications than other groups; they are more likely to have multiple physical health problems and die prematurely. It is unlikely that this profile of health and social inequalities is so uniformly and globally poor due to the stigmatising behaviours of individual actors and institutions.

The onset of schizophrenia occurs at a crucial time in the young person's life, with devastating consequences to relationships, educational and occupational opportunities. At a time when young people are amidst the often-challenging management of identity, sexuality and career, the disruption caused by psychotic symptoms is immense. Narrowly defined, schizophrenia is marked by having delusions and pronounced hallucinations, and where the person lacks any insight as to the origins of these hallucinations. More broadly defined, the person experiencing a psychotic episode will exhibit disorganised behaviours and speech that are sometimes incomprehensible. Additionally, pharmacological treatments intended to suppress hallucinations, have several characteristics that interfere with and alter the physical health, personality, and social skills of the person. The medication may produce physiological changes – lethargy, weight gain; the person may experience restlessness and agitation. Commonly, there is an impact on appearance – a neglect of personal hygiene and clothing. The severity of the symptoms, positive or negative, is likely to be detrimental to any meaningful engagement with others. Finding employment or returning to education may not be a priority for anyone trapped in a psychotic illness and, even when the symptoms subside due to medication, the physical and psychological resources required to resume a 'normal' life trajectory may be too depleted for this to be realised.

Stigma as discriminatory behaviour on the part of employing organisations, therefore, cannot satisfactorily account for the high levels of unemployment among people with schizophrenia. A more likely source is the debilitating effects of the illness on a wide range of personal resources and skills. Of course, companies and management *do* discriminate against people known or perceived to have mental health problems but this more likely to happen to people with common mental disorders such as depression. That is, employers may anticipate, possibly based on stereotype, that the person will lack the competencies or skills to undertake the role effectively. While we should not confuse the concepts of trust and *confidence*, here the semantic connection between the two is strong. We have noted that vulnerability must play a role, otherwise trust is irrelevant. Intuitively one is likely to conclude that the vulnerability resides with the person with the mental health problem. However, the structures of most organisations are such that there are obvious liabilities for supervisors too, should they appoint someone who fails to deliver or causes a problem within the organisation. Motivations may be multiple and complex. The manager may be motivated by either, or a combination of experience, prejudice, clash of personality and self-interest. Nevertheless, we know that while disabilities and equal rights legislation may be in place to protect against work-related discrimination, these are difficult to police, especially for the often-hidden disability in mental illness.

Returning to the experience of people with a psychosis whose symptoms are somewhat more visible, the evidence suggests that employment opportunities are highly restricted, and associated with individual factors including lower cognitive and social functioning, greater levels of negative and depressive symptoms and poor educational attainment (Tandberg et al., 2013). While there are few good longitudinal studies of employment and severe mental illness, findings from a Swedish register population (Holm et al., 2021) showed that a quarter of people later diagnosed with a psychosis had been employed, highlighting the likely prodromal difficulties emerging in adolescence. Five years later, the proportion of people employed, dropped to 10%. The key factors associated with post-employment diagnosis were educational attainment, older age at diagnosis, no substance use, marriage or cohabitation, and few hospitalisations, suggesting that such individuals were functioning quite well and had social support. Other evidence suggests that lifetime unemployment is related to the level of impairments experienced (Harvey et al., 2012) and that those with a less chronic course showed substantial improvements throughout their working life (Hakulinen et al., 2019).

Again, while the evidence of extremely low rates of employment among people with severe mental illness is incontrovertible, much less in known about employment-seeking and discrimination in this population. Certainly, some of the low and deteriorating employment can be explained by medical and social factors described in the studies above but may also be attributed to the vagaries of welfare and disability benefits which disincentivise job-seeking among this population (Kirsh, 2016). However, it is also true that feelings of low self-worth inhibit ambition and block change for most people, let alone people with diagnosed mental health conditions.

Anticipated stigma and agency

Trust has cognitive dimensions of course – thoughts, knowledge, memory – but the emotional aspects as noted in the discussion on childhood and attachment, play an important role too. Indeed, the distinction between cognition and feelings is somewhat false in that they don't operate on distinctly separate areas of the brain to the extent that affect may be necessary for normal conscious experience, language fluency, and memory (Duncan & Barrett, 2007). Feelings inform actions. The feelings generated by an experience play a large part in determining either repeat exposure or avoidance. People with a mental illness of any sort, commonly experience low self-esteem – they may regard themselves somewhere on a negative spectrum, from not very competent to a truly malign entity. They may have grown up with these feelings of worthlessness, predisposing them to mental health problems, or acquired them as part of the illness experience. Their low self-esteem provokes a generalised mistrust of their own capacity to function appropriately in social situations, and mistrust of social response to their presence. Whatever, the origins of such feelings, many mentally ill people radically censor their potential social worlds in anticipation of failure or rejection in the public gaze. The concept of self-stigma is relatively new (Watson et al., 2007). While public stigma concerns the negative attitudes held by people and communities, self-stigma is the internalisation of these beliefs and attitudes, and these are reinforced by associated behaviours. One theoretical model about the process of internalisation, contends that a person with severe mental illness must first be aware of the negative public beliefs about the qualities and propensities associated with mental illness, then agree with these beliefs. In the final stage of the process, the individual begins to apply the negative public appraisal to him- or herself (Corrigan et al., 2009). In a modified account of labelling theory, Scheff (2017) explains how an individual (or group) on receipt of a particular label or categorisation, may often begin to assume the assigned identity and behave in ways that undermine what should be their self-interests. In this model people with severe mental illness internalise the low expectations, perceived or otherwise, of others. Again, poor-self-esteem creates social 'invisibility' and less agency in the self-determination of personal needs which consequently impact on health behaviours and poor physical health.

Whitehead et al.'s (2016) synthesis of theories and causal pathways connecting the level of control in the living environment to disparities in health outcomes for people with severe and enduring mental illness is relevant to this doubly disadvantaged population. Thus, Charlton and White (1995) suggest that access to resources, offset by needs, results in an individual's 'margin of resources' the size of which predicts social position, level of inequality, and consequently their level of control and autonomy within different social positions. Along with 'time preference' these factors influence health-related behaviours and access to services, etc. 'Time preference' here indicates the degree to which an individual can invest their resources in an uncertain future. In this context, disadvantaged groups (e.g., low income, severe mental illness) choose immediately available rewards (present time preference), rather than unspecified future gains. Present time preferences, as is often the case of people living with mental illness, are linked to unhealthy, sugar-rich diets, alcohol and cigarette use, and inactive lifestyles, despite the anticipation of their future health damaging effects. Despite the potential for recovery models of care, our work among service users highlights a vicious circle of stigma, low-self-esteem, poor diet, smoking, and fatalism. Whitehead and colleagues argue that control, autonomy, and power to exercise choice help facilitate access to resources to promote and maintain health and agree with Sen (2014) that relative low autonomy and powerlessness underpins and maintains socio-economic and health inequalities.

Social networks and friendships

While much of the literature on stigma tends to concern social attitudes, there is little understanding of the experiences of people with a mental illness (Rose et al., 2011). The closure of the large asylums in the late 20th century and the relocation of patients with chronic mental health problems into the community did not result in a fluid dispersal of such people into family homes and individual private rented accommodation but rather, a new stratum of organised healthcare based on different levels of supported housing monitored by community mental health teams (psychiatry, nursing, and social work). This was a sensible and pragmatic approach to rehousing many thousands of people and ensuring some level of healthcare and rehabilitation. In many cities there are clusters of people with long-term conditions living in shared accommodation – mini-institutions containing people who become reliant upon each other and the volunteers sometimes connected to professional support teams. In countries with no or sub-optimal welfare, increasing numbers of mentally ill people are homeless.

While acknowledging that social networks are important for health and well-being, generally, low self-esteem and diminished expectations of life can be reflected, amplified, and reinforced by people in the same social networks. Thus, social networks may provide social supports as buffers against the health-limiting stressors but can also influence and reinforce negative health behaviours through harmful beliefs normatively held by the group. In a landmark study, Christakis and colleagues' work (Christakis & Fowler, 2007) on networks and weight found clusters of obesity which couldn't be attributable to the selective development of social ties among similarly obese persons but rather, that obesity 'spread' by connection. Thus, an individual's chances of becoming obese increased significantly whatever their relationship. A later study showed similar results for cigarette smoking and cessation, the authors indicating that close and distant social ties influence smoking behaviour, and that groups of interconnected people also cease smoking together (Christakis & Fowler, 2008). While the impact of social connectedness may be overstated in some studies (Ehsan et al., 2019), the importance of group or peer influences on all types of behaviour is clear. Intuitively, we trust those who are in a similar position to ourselves.[5] For people with severe mental health problems, the influence of 'peers' on health and other behaviours may require additional consideration. First, people with severe mental illness have smaller friendship networks than other people generally (Cohen & Sokolovsky, 1978), and that network size decreases over the course of the illness (Palumbo et al., 2015). Worse still, the evidence suggests that family members account for most the network size in this population.[6] In our own work, service users had similarly restricted networks and mostly comprised of people who attended the same day centre or lived with them in sheltered accommodation. Poor diet and heavy smoking in their 'group' homes were highly prevalent, as was the consumption of many litres of sugary drinks. Many had picked up these behaviours from long spells in psychiatric hospitals, where the 'sharing' of unhealthy goods supported friendship networks; a kind of institutional behaviour, it was not discarded in the community.

Social exclusion

With considerable variation in quality and quantity, most communities have cultural or natural 'assets' such as libraries, arts and music venues, or parks; places that most people can access and appreciate. People with severe mental illness often describe extreme loneliness and exclusion in their daily lives, partially attributing this to the shame and hurt arising from public hostility and rejection. As part of a recent project (Leavey, 2023) on social exclusion, participants reported that they no longer visited public venues because they worried about 'having a breakdown', and anticipated being unable to deal with the reactions of other people. Strikingly, while most people had experienced micro-aggressions from other people, avoidance is provoked by a profound self-consciousness of being gazed at by other people as though mental illness was obviously exhibited in clothes or physical appearance. These are not delusions in the strictest meaning, so despite a degree of obvious reflexivity, an understanding that their fears may be groundless, they remain trapped by their fears. Here, the term trapped can be used either as *confinement,* or *being tricked or deceived into doing something contrary to their own interests.* Again, while the threats to one's safety and wellbeing may be more perceived than real, the habitus – in this case an avoidance strategy engrained over years, reinforces the desire for confinement, however miserable, because it is predictable.

> I remember going to the shop by myself and I used to leave the basket at the door and the trolley wherever and walk out, I couldn't do it. My depression was so bad, and anxiety was so bad it just couldn't even stay there run the shop stand in a queue or anything… It was just complete fear. And I thought everyone was looking at me and all this which obviously wasn't true, but I felt it was true.
>
> (Anne)

> Anywhere familiar, I can go by myself. Any new places? I can't do it. There's just way too much. I mean, I've struggled to mow my front grass, due to my perception that the neighbours are all watching me. Because you know, I don't get out there often. I don't socialize with the neighbours too much. So, I presume that they think I'm a sort of weird loner sort of guy; you know, keep myself to myself.
>
> (Jack)

Importantly however, many participants described past interests and retained hope of reconnecting with these. While there are often a wide range of activities that are available within voluntary and community organisations these tend to be 'in-house' rather than 'in-community'. In this sense, the trust that people with mental illness have for such organisations is created by well-meaning routinisation which offers security but at the cost of paralysis in growth and exclusion from other community-based activities. Although feeling safe in day-centres, they acknowledge the reinforcement of stigma and separation. This dependency on fixed provision also means that this population's needs choices are restricted to the centres' availability and therefore they often remain isolated in their accommodation at evenings, weekends, and public holidays. The additional benefits of friendships and peer support within the centres are unavailable when the centres are closed. Service users also described their attachment to individual centre staff. While such individuals are often inspiring and helpful, their departure creates a loss of tacit knowledge with discontinuities of resources and trust. Community organisations are aware of these challenges but appear 'stuck' within an outdated model of support while funding continues to be based on buildings and attendance but lacking any evaluation of outcomes related to social inclusion and health improvement.

The challenges posed by public stigma and self-stigma are compounded by the general 'invisibility' of this group to those who provide and manage community assets, possibly explained by a knowledge deficit about severe mental illness. Although our discussions with community asset providers (e.g., local authorities, Sports, Arts, and green spaces) revealed an awareness about anxiety and depression, they knew nothing about the physical health and mortality of people with severe mental illness. Significantly, while other health-related disabilities are acknowledged in policy, processes, and public information, severe mental illness is absent. Moreover, we noted that this knowledge gap is also true for many of the community and voluntary sector agencies. What is clear is that there are multiple and interacting personal and social processes that erect barriers to the local community resources, not just access to the labour market, that most people take for granted. Graham Thornicroft, an eminent psychiatrist and campaigner against stigma in mental illness, argues that while there is scant evidence about what types of interventions are useful in reducing stigma in its various manifestations and context, the profound impact of the media in fostering grossly harmful misinformation about mental illness, exhibiting prejudices that would not be acceptable if used against other sectors of the population (Thornicroft et al., 2016). Human rights approaches and legislation to tackle discrimination and prejudice may be required.

Notes

1 At its most basic, power is played out in numbers, and the distribution of rights and resources is often based on one's position within social hierarchies or in Marxian terms, one's relationship to the means of production. The latter's hard materialist position also asserts that the norms and values of any society will be that of the ruling classes. While the identification of a single entity called the 'ruling class' is unlikely due to the plurality and complexity of post-modern societies, the symbolic boundaries that signify class positions and interests are still discernible, albeit more blurred than those a century ago.

2 This is not unique to jews, of course. From an Irish background herself, Douglas noted the continuation of eating fish on Fridays among Irish migrants in England long after the changes brought about by Vatican ii, reinforced a boundary between them and their English neighbours.

3 While Severe Mental Illness (SMI) tends to be defined as consisting of three criteria: a psychiatric diagnosis (either DSM or ICD), illness duration of more than 2 years, and disability in functioning, it is commonly understood to be a psychotic disorder (e.g., schizophrenia) or bi-polar disorder. Other researchers include major depressive disorder due to its duration and impact on functioning.

4 In 2022, Ms Hutchinson, a 26-year-old former Whitehouse assistant who became a critical witness in the Senate Committee hearings on the January 6th riots at the Capital buildings, was subjected to vilification on social media by the ex-president and his followers 'as a girl' with 'serious problems' – 'mental problems'. As the *New York Times* reported at time, the former President has often publicly treated women who challenge him, criticising them in personal terms intending to call into question their credibility, sanity, and self-worth.

5 Retail and advertising organisations spend generous sums of money on the basis that it is easier to trust (and, thus buy from) representatives (actors) in the same social class, age group, or gender.

6 Anecdotally, psychiatric service users commonly report their keyworkers as part of their friendship network, which of course, is a misrecognition of the relationship.

References

Bourdieu, P. (1977). *Outline of a theory of practice*. Cambridge University Press.

Charlton, B. G., & White, M. (1995). Living on the margin: A salutogenic model for socio-economic differentials in health. *Public Health, 109*(4), 235–243. https://doi.org/10.1016/s0033-3506(95)80200-2

Christakis, N. A., & Fowler, J. H. (2007). The spread of obesity in a large social network over 32 years. *The New England Journal of Medicine, 357*(4), 370–379. https://doi.org/10.1056/NEJMsa066082

Christakis, N. A., & Fowler, J. H. (2008). The collective dynamics of smoking in a large social network. *The New England Journal of Medicine, 358*(21), 2249–2258. https://doi.org/10.1056/NEJMsa0706154

Cohen, C. I., & Sokolovsky, J. (1978). Schizophrenia and social networks: Ex-patients in the inner city. *Schizophrenia Bulletin, 4*(4), 546–560. https://doi.org/10.1093/schbul/4.4.546

Corrigan, P. W., Bink, A. B., Schmidt, A., Jones, N., & Rüsch, N. (2016). What is the impact of self-stigma? Loss of self-respect and the "why try" effect. *Journal of Mental Health, 25*(1), 10–15.

Corrigan, P. W., Larson, J. E., & Rüsch, N. (2009). Self-stigma and the "why try" effect: Impact on life goals and evidence-based practices. *World Psychiatry, 8*(2), 75–81. https://doi.org/10.1002/j.2051-5545.2009.tb00218.x

Corrigan, P. W., Mueser, K. T., Bond, G. R., Drake, R. E., & Solomon, P. (2008). *Principles and practices of psychiatric rehabilitation: An empirical approach*. Guilford Press.

Douglas, M. (2002). *Purity and danger*. Routledge.

Duncan, S., & Barrett, L. F. (2007). Affect is a form of cognition: A neurobiological analysis. *Cognition and Emotion, 21*(6), 1184–1211. https://doi.org/10.1080/02699930701437931

Ehsan, A., Klaas, H. S., Bastianen, A., & Spini, D. (2019). Social capital and health: A systematic review of systematic reviews. *SSM Population Health, 8*, 100425. https://doi.org/10.1016/j.ssmph.2019.100425

Foucault, M. (1977). *Madness & civilization: A history of insanity in the age of reason.* Tavistock Publications.

Goffman, E. (1963). *Stigma: Notes on the management of a spoiled identity.* Prentice Hall.

Hakulinen, C., McGrath, J. J., Timmerman, A., Skipper, N., Mortensen, P. B., Pedersen, C. B., & Agerbo, E. (2019). The association between early-onset schizophrenia with employment, income, education, and cohabitation status: Nationwide study with 35 years of follow-up. *Social Psychiatry and Psychiatric Epidemiology, 54*(11), 1343–1351. https://doi.org/10.1007/s00127-019-01756-0

Harvey, P. D., Heaton, R. K., Carpenter, W. T. Jr., Green, M. F., Gold, J. M., & Schoenbaum, M. (2012). Functional impairment in people with schizophrenia: Focus on employability and eligibility for disability compensation. *Schizophrenia Research, 140*(1-3), 1–8. https://doi.org/10.1016/j.schres.2012.03.025

Holm, M., Taipale, H., Tanskanen, A., Tiihonen, J., & Mitterdorfer-Rutz, E. (2021). Employment among people with schizophrenia or bipolar disorder: A population-based study using nationwide registers. *Acta Psychiatrica Scandinavica, 143*(1), 61–71. https://doi.org/10.1111/acps.13254

Jorm, A. F. (2000). Mental health literacy: Public knowledge and beliefs about mental disorders. *British Journal of Psychiatry, 177*, 396–401. https://www.bjp.rcpsych.org/ http:www.rcpsych.ac.uk

Killaspy, H. (2006). From the asylum to community care: Learning from experience. *British Medical Bulletin, 79-80*, 245–258. https://doi.org/10.1093/bmb/ldl017

Kirmayer, L. J., & Robbins, J. M. (1996). Patients who somatize in primary care: A longitudinal study of cognitive and social characteristics. *Psychological Medicine, 26*, 937–951.

Kirsh, B. (2016). Client, contextual and program elements influencing supported employment: A literature review. *Community Mental Health Journal, 52*(7), 809–820. https://doi.org/10.1007/s10597-015-9936-7

Leavey, G. (2023). *Challenging health outcomes - Integrated caring environments (CHOICE).* Ulster University. https://www.ulster.ac.uk/research/topic/psychology/projects/choice

Leavey, G., Rosato, M., Galway, K., Hughes, L., Mallon, S., & Rondon, J. (2016). Patterns and predictors of help seeking contacts with health services and general practice detection of suicidality. *BMC Psychiatry, 16*(1), 120.

Link, B. G., & Phelan, J. (2014). Stigma power. *Social Science & Medicine, 103*, 24–32. https://doi.org/10.1016/j.socscimed.2013.07.035

Palumbo, C., Volpe, U., Matanov, A., Priebe, S., & Giacco, D. (2015). Social networks of patients with psychosis: A systematic review. *BMC Research Notes, 8*, 560. https://doi.org/10.1186/s13104-015-1528-7

Patel, V., Saxena, S., Lund, C., Thornicroft, G., Baingana, F., Bolton, P., Chisholm, D., Collins, P. Y., Cooper, J. L., Eaton, J., Herrman, H., Herzallah, M. M., Huang, Y., Jordans, M. J. D., Kleinman, A., Medina-Mora, M. E., Morgan, E., Niaz, U., Omigbodun, O., ... UnÜtzer, J. (2018). The Lancet Commission on global mental health and sustainable development. *The Lancet, 392*(10157), 1553–1598. https://doi.org/10.1016/S0140-6736(18)31612-X

Rosendal, M., Oleson, F., & Fink, P. (2005). Management of medically unexplained symptoms. *British Medical Journal, 330*, 4–5.

Rose, D., Willis, R., Brohan, E., Sartorius, N., Villiares, C., & Thornicroft, G. (2011). Reported stigma and discrimination by people with a diagnosis of schizophrenia. *Epidemiology and Psychiatric Sciences, 20*, 193–204.

Scheff, T. J. (2017). *Being mentally ill: A sociological study.* Routledge.

Sen, A. (2014). Development as freedom (1999). In *The globalization and development reader: perspectives on development and global change* (p. 525). Alfred A. Knopf, Inc.

Tandberg, M., Sundet, K., Andreassen, O. A., Melle, I., & Ueland, T. (2013). Occupational functioning, symptoms and neurocognition in patients with psychotic disorders: Investigating subgroups based on social security status. *Social Psychiatry and Psychiatric Epidemiology*, *48*(6), 863–874. https://doi.org/10.1007/s00127-012-0598-2

Thornicroft, G., Mehta, N., Clement, S., Evans-Lacko, S., Doherty, M., Rose, D., Koschorke, M., Shidhaye, R., O'Reilly, C., & Henderson, C. (2016). Evidence for effective interventions to reduce mental-health-related stigma and discrimination. *Lancet*, *387*(10023), 1123–1132. https://doi.org/10.1016/s0140-6736(15)00298-6

Watson, A. C., Corrigan, P., Larson, J. E., & Sells, M. (2007). Self-stigma in people with mental illness. *Schizophrenia Bulletin*, *33*(6), 1312–1318. https://doi.org/10.1093/schbul/sbl076

Whitehead, M., Pennington, A., Orton, L., Nayak, S., Petticrew, M., Sowden, A., & White, M. (2016). How could differences in 'control over destiny' lead to socio-economic inequalities in health? A synthesis of theories and pathways in the living environment. *Health & Place*, *39*, 51–61. https://doi.org/10.1016/j.healthplace.2016.02.002

Chapter 10

Conclusion

Madness in various forms has probably always existed. Our histories are full of people deemed irrational, regarded by fellow citizens as eccentric, or exhibiting beliefs and behaviours that didn't quite fit in with the expectations of the community. Many people experience 'mental health problems' and many more people have been in direct contact with someone who has, as either a friend, family member, lover, or work colleague. Confessional media platforms regularly give voice to people who unashamedly claim to have experienced a mental illness, almost a badge of honour. Conversely, the employment of mental illness in the cause of dishonour is commonplace – for example, 'accusations' of mental illness made as part of political campaigns to reduce an opponent's presentation of competence and trustworthiness.

Beliefs about the origins of mental illness, whether determined by social, biological, or even supernatural, matter because they tell us something about the dominance and direction of scientific and philosophical forces in a given society while offering distinct directions for the recognition, management, treatment, and care of individuals designated as having this or that type of disorder. In some cultures, those considered as different were offered a special place in the community, as highly spiritual, possessing insights and visions not available to others; in other societies, such people were rejected by the community, deemed too unpredictable to have a productive role, to have value. In many parts of the world today people who do not live or love in the way that their societies or politicians demand can be incarcerated or murdered. Mostly those who experience a mental illness are simply denied recognition and are excluded from most areas of social life and activity.

I have tried to show that mental disorders have a genetic and a social basis, some people are more vulnerable than others not just because of their biology but by social circumstances and events, by the actions and inactions of others that impinge upon and distort the individual's sense of reality. The loss of trust and often the misplacement of trust in others are among the greatest casualties of individual and social 'breakdown' providing the basis for disruption, estrangement, and loneliness. People with mental disorders are likely to become marginalised and excluded, while marginalised and excluded people become vulnerable to mental disorders. In the intrapsychic and interpersonal worlds of those who experience

DOI: 10.4324/9781003326687-10

trauma or schizophrenia, or simply cut off from others, existential and ontological trust can often dissolve, leaving uncertainty and mistrust about reality and their own place within it. For example, those who experience post-traumatic stress disorder (PTSD) are altered in their interpersonal relations but are also transformed biologically and in relationship to themselves. That symptoms and behaviours subsumed under the general rubric of a mental illness require any kind of response is an acknowledgement that they are not just a problem for the individual, but also to family and society.

Throughout this book the concept of the stranger will have been witnessed. It is an apt description of how society views and responds to mental illness but also the ways in which we create boundaries to establish the status of the stranger and the beliefs and behaviours that are judged to be perplexing and/or unacceptable. Even, perhaps especially, within families the individual with a mental illness is often considered symbolically lost and no longer the 'self' that they once were, they become 'strangers'. Simultaneously, they are recognisable but unfamiliar and untrustworthy. As an aspect of epistemic injustice (Carel & Kidd, 2014), the views of people with mental health problems are disparaged or simply ignored through the designation and power of stigma in various forms and guises (Sakakibara, 2023). The consequences of this injustice are not only evident in the social exclusion of this population but in premature death from preventable causes.

There are several challenges in conceptualising trust in the relationship between a mental health professional and the detention of someone with a severe mental illness. With severe cognitive impairment, for example in those with dementia or the impaired mental capacity of someone experiencing a psychotic episode, the barriers to trust-building between patients and clinicians are significant. Does the concept of trust even apply in such cases? Moreover, resistance to a psychiatric diagnosis is pivotal. While a medical diagnosis often brings relief to those experiencing symptoms, a psychiatric diagnosis is seldom welcomed, a problem that is amplified by historical intersectional factors of race and social class. The rejection of psychiatry by people who may benefit from treatment, and the potential for coercive approaches to assessment and hospitalisation undermines the building of trust relations with the institution. Unlike general medical care, hospital admission and treatment may require arrangements made with family members and without the individual's consent, police and physical force may be used. Additionally, factors related to ethnicity and class often complicates engagement through a combination of systemic cultural ignorance and discriminatory beliefs and practices, producing alienation with services and relatively poor patient outcomes. Thus, trust-building between patients and mental healthcare professionals is undermined by structural violence, the racial discrimination, and the historical mistreatment of minoritised groups, inside mental health services, and social institutions more generally.

For over 30 years, psychiatry in the United Kingdom and the United States has been forced to respond to criticism about the treatment of young black people in the mental health system. Central to this debate has been the misdiagnosis and overrepresentation of this population among people who have been involuntarily detained in psychiatric units, a situation worsened by the use of police in its undertaking. In many instances, such detentions have occurred with varying degrees of violence. The deaths of young black men with signs of mental illness while in police custody have added to the perception of that the mental health system and the police collude in the brutalisation and murder of black people. Again, these perceptions are reinforced by the additional overrepresentation of black people in the forensic mental health system, where the boundaries between controlled criminal detention and therapeutic care and control are somewhat blurred. Often commented upon but mostly supported by anecdotal evidence, is the degree to which the dynamics of detention-resistance violence is propelled by a stereotyped belief among hospital staff that young black men are inherently violent. Their response to resistance is often disproportionate force, the product of self-fulfilling prophecy. While much has been done to improve mental health services for black and minority ethnic patients, the seminal determinants of conflict lie outside the boundaries of the healthcare system.

Much remains to be done within healthcare in terms of education and training health professionals to be culturally competent practitioners so that misdiagnosis and inappropriate responses to suffering are minimalised. However, providing culturally competent services although needed, merely scratches the surface of pathogenic social structures. Galtung's concept of structural violence has been developed further as a way of addressing institutionalised health inequalities through improving the *structural competency* of healthcare professionals (Metzl & Hansen, 2018) through which the social, political, and economic determinants of physical and mental illnesses are recognised by clinicians and, in doing so can be incorporated in treatment and care plans. What is being advocated is a major shift in the medical gaze and the transcendence of traditional medical boundaries to incorporate understanding of the power structures that produce patient health beliefs and behaviours, the conditions and circumstances that give rise to the challenges that are often dismissed as aspects of pathology or maladaptive cultures. In part too, this approach demands that clinicians begin to examine their own privileged position within the social structure and how the management of mental health problems will require public health approaches and structural change.

The anomalous nature of the mentally ill in our society is also projected onto the professional systems designated to manage mental illness. If general medicine is typically regarded as trustworthy, this esteem seems much less true for psychiatry, strangely so, given the prominence of mental illness in public policy and funding.[1] Despite the ubiquity and cost of mental illness, among the general public and even other branches of medicine there is a suspicion of inauthenticity about psychiatry that those who practice it, aren't 'really doctors'. Of course, in popular culture, 'real' doctors deal with diseased organs and broken limbs, they dash magnificently – they cure people or when they can't, they speak comfortingly to grieving relatives. This is not the world of psychiatry and mental health services. While people with neuroses or phobias can be helped to return to healthy functioning, our scientific understanding of the origins of schizophrenia remains obscure placing the possibility of a cure as a distant aspiration.

Psychiatry's own struggle for identity as a scientific enterprise has for many years left the institution vacillating between analysis of the mind or examination of the brain in the search for the origins of our troubles. The often-futile attempts at organic and pharmaceutical rearranging of the brain left much human destruction and mistrust of the profession in its wake. Alternatively, the reconstruction of mind and the significance of indelible childhood memories established by Freud and his followers remain largely outside the public's grasp, and however beneficial it may be to those who can obtain it, is often the subject of scepticism inside and outside the profession. Presenting the appearance of trustworthiness is often problematic in the context of internal conflict and uncertainty. However, trust in the profession is much more complicated in that those who may *need* help, are often those who don't want it, either at all or not in the way that it is offered. As described in previous chapters, the individual's explanatory model of his problem may not fit with psychiatry's model in which case he may feel threatened and distrustful of what is being offered in psychiatric services. Alternatively, he may not have any explanation for what he is experiencing but doesn't want any kind of help and/or does not wish anyone to know that he has mental health problems. As noted in previous chapters, the psychiatric profession and psychiatric hospital care are vicariously stigmatised, a historical, often imagined as a gloomy malign presence.

Finding solutions

We are regularly warned that aging populations and shrinking economies require innovative approaches to healthcare, solutions that increasingly seem technical and non-human. Modernity, expressed in highly complex and abstract systems of connection and communication appears increasingly remote, unaccountable, and unpredictable – demanding new forms of trust or possibly just resigned acceptance. Possibly unanticipated by Giddens in the 1990s when his perspectives on trust were written, the demand for technological solutions to an extraordinary range of human activities and needs including economic, health, cultural, and educational. Competitive, economic-driven policy enthusiasm for technology either fails to acknowledge or simply wilfully ignores its long-term negative consequences. By the time these potential outcomes are more widely understood, the seeds have already germinated with profoundly negative consequences for social conflict, the source of much suffering. They may also be less helpful in assisting therapeutic care than governments imagine. Thus, while digital technology may facilitate exchange and participation there is alarm at the propensity for new technology such as artificial intelligence (AI) to manufacture disinformation and divisive manipulation. Trust in institutional systems and interpersonal trust depends on the quality and level of information between and within communities, and between individuals, and government, particularly where perspectives diverge. Thus, communities and individuals may differ in their visions for society but should have equal access to the same 'facts'. In healthcare interventions, generative AI promises rapid detection of disease, much more efficiently than humans. The vast amounts of information generated by AI in multiple formats appear intelligent but lack thought and feeling. AI models often produce wrong outputs, prone to what the computing researchers describe as 'hallucination', drifting into fabulous, non-sensical and misleading content (Monteith et al., 2024). Although AI models are potentially beneficial for health care in terms of rapid and accurate testing, screening, and the development of pharmaceuticals and vaccines, they also generate outputs which reproduce social prejudices, and information that is dangerously incorrect. The pace of AI innovation appears to be outstripping our ethical frameworks for understanding and regulating the new technologies, and institutional policy on trust and safeguarding.

When trust is thin or absent, the activities between agents are tightly regulated. However, despite current alarm about the dangers of social media and AI, policy-makers seem to be in a state of paralysis as to how to respond to the direction of digital expansion and its impact on society and the individual. The evidence thus far on the impact of the internet and social media on trust and mental health is often ambivalent but veering towards a general public alarm on the damage done to children and adolescents. If our actions, self-esteem, and relationships, to name a few, are shaped and directed by beliefs and knowledge, then trustworthy information in the development of wellbeing is clearly important. For now, a plausibly significant connection between sanity and digital media trust lies in a seemingly unrestrained capacity of digital platforms used by all kinds of actors to convey vast amounts of unfiltered and unregulated knowledge and information across boundaryless societies and communities. While this communication flow may have an obvious liberating attractiveness and efficiency, governments and citizens, albeit for different reasons, are only recently alert to the dangers created by untrustworthy and malevolent actors. The substitution of human 'customer service' employees, counsellors, therapists and teachers, to name a few professions, with machine-learning chatbots promises substantial economic benefits to corporations but can be a major source of stress to people forced to seek help from them. It is generally the case that most people don't trust the *new technology* but are left with no choice.[2] While the absence of communication with a responsible human entity to resolve problems that arise from services and goods are stressful, concerns about the internet and social media's influence on the mental health of children, particularly, have intensified.

However, if trust 'happens' in the absence of information, what kind of information is available, and provided by whom and when, matters significantly. In relation to help-seeking and psychiatric services, vast, continually expanding amounts of evidence-free health 'information, advice, treatments, and services' are available for emotional and psychological problems, many of which are silly, exploitative, or harmful. In conditions of mistrust in psychiatry and psychiatric services or where there are long-waiting lists for treatment, the internet provides a responsive marketplace but one that is largely unpoliced and unaccountable. Also linked to the scarcity of publicly funded mental health services, there is considerable interest by governments and a commensurate investment in the use of 'chatbots',

AI-generated computer programs, to deliver counselling services to young people (Gratzer & Goldbloom, 2019). While these may be attractive to people disinclined to seek help, the possibility of trust-building in abstract algorithms remains dubious. In any case, there is no evidence currently that chatbots as a substitute for human contact and advice are effective or desirable.

Dissolving distance and familiarisation

How does a clinician obtain the trust of patient who are appear so withdrawn that they are unable to connect with anyone? The psychiatrist and psychoanalyst Anthony Bateman and colleagues (2000, p. 67) suggest that

> Seeking help from a stranger is bound to arouse anxieties and provoke conflicts additional to any already underlying a patient's symptoms. Will he understand? Will he be able to help? Will he want to help me? Will he think I am wasting his time? Will he judge me harshly as too bad or too mad to be helped? The patient's wish to protect himself from the dangers implicit in questions such as these can conflict with his intention to be honest. Reticence and mistrust at interview exist over and above unconscious defence mechanisms …How the therapist meets the patient and responds to his tentative approaches helps to determine whether the patient feels the necessary initial trust.

These questions reflect the patients' anxieties, commonly imbued with additional reflexive concerns related to identity whether, gender, ethnicity or class, about how they will be perceived by the psychiatrist. The cognitive-based structural and cultural competencies discussed previously require supplementary affective skills, those that transcend the objective professional distance ('affective neutrality'). To obtain patients' trust requires a transcendence of professionalism beyond the rigidities of managerialism, out of which the clinician demonstrates authenticity and compassion.

Arthur Kleinman (1988) describes in raw and unflinching detail, his experience as a young medical student charged with attending to the needs of a young girl with severe burns that covered most of her body. 'She had to undergo the ordeal of a whirlpool bath during which the burnt flesh was tweezered away'. His job was to hold her uninjured hand. 'Clumsily with a beginner's uncertainty of how to proceed, I tried to distract this little patient from her traumatic daily confrontation with terrible pain. I tried talking to her about her home, her family, her school – almost anything that might draw her vigilant attention away from her suffering. I could barely tolerate the daily horror: her screams, dead tissue floating in the blood-stained water, the peeling flesh, the oozing wounds, the battles over cleaning and bandaging. Then one day, I made contact. At wit's end, angered at my own ignorance and impotence, uncertain what to besides clutching the small hand, and in despair over her unrelenting anguish, I found myself asking her to tell me how she tolerated it, what the feeling was like of being so badly burned and having to experience the awful surgical ritual, day after day. She stopped, quite surprised, and looked at me from a face so disfigured it was difficult to read the expression; then, in terms direct and simple, she told me. While she spoke, she grasped my hand harder and neither screamed not fought off the surgeon or the nurse. Each day, from then on, her trust established, she tried to give me a feeling of what she was experiencing'. Kleinman tells the reader that by the time he had left the unit, the girl was much better at managing her treatment and pain, and that he had gained from her a valuable lesson 'that it is possible to talk with patients, even those who are most distressed, about the actual experience of illness, and that witnessing and helping to order that experience can be of therapeutic value'.

Kleinman's work throughout his lifetime tells us something important about illness, suffering and the human condition. Kleinman's narratives illustrate the distinction between the clinician's attention to disease and the body, and the patient's experience of illness but as in the story of the suffering child, they also speak to the importance of compassion in medicine in the building of trust and therapeutic engagement. Every aspect of the child's being, from her distressing appearance and screams, might convey the sense of being an alien to most people and provoke, as they did in Kleinman, a desire to retreat to someone and something more comfortable. That someone was able to seek an understanding of the other's suffering in the high stakes of profound intimacy, permitted a bridge to trust and then to healing that had not hitherto existed. I refer to the high stakes of profound intimacy because for patient and clinician there is considerable vulnerability on both sides. Kleinman took a gamble to stray from the comfort zone of tedious but presumably expected questions about home and school which must have sounded to her as both patronising and stupefying, social worlds a million light years from the child's current excruciating and existential predicament. By seeking to know more about the trauma and how she experienced it, allowed him to bear witness to something present and real, rather than exacerbate her suffering. For the child, the authenticity of Kleinman's engagement with his own empathic humanity permitted a willingness to confide her own truths and vulnerability. These intimate spaces create a levelling up of power between doctor and patient the possibility of authentic trust.

Authenticity and trust

The projection of authenticity by healthcare professionals as a foundational block of trust-building is manifested in specific behaviours (Cook et al., 2004), best described as person-centred approaches which acknowledge the personal dimensions of the patient, extending the boundaries of physician interest to the experience of illness. The themes that emerged in our exploration of trust and help-seeking, young people described feeling 'unseen', almost literally, when their physician made no eye contact with them when taking notes and then appeared to rush through the encounter to write a prescription without first getting to know the person, their situation, and their preferences for treatment. Bear in mind that young adolescents approach their first direct family doctor consultation with trepidation having previously been accompanied by a parent. In many ways, family doctors are also 'strangers' to whom they may have to confide information about their bodies, sexuality and mental health, experiences and emotions that are often concealed from parents and friends. In these encounters, they feel exposed and vulnerable during consultations with people much older, may be of the opposite sex and often from a different social and cultural milieu. While some of the criticisms and anxieties expressed about the family doctor can appear unfounded and perhaps exaggerated, the mistrust tends to emanate from the young person's lack of connection with doctors. If trust is a bridge to an anticipated positive outcome, mistrust is a barrier to such outcomes based on uncertainty that can be disassembled through authentic interaction, from face-to-face communication rather than mediated knowledge that may be generated elsewhere.[3]

The demand for health services are such that the ability of family doctors to provide adequate time for patients to feel comfortable and confident about describing intimate contextual details about the possible origins of failing mental health, and thus, what the potential remedies might be. Where these are social in origin, as they often are, pharmaceutical treatment may simply dampen symptoms, rather than remove the source of the problem. When patients feel that they are not 'properly listened to' by physicians, or feel that they are being patronised, trust is eroded or failing in its construction. A study of adherence to anti-depressant use found that less than a fifth of patients maintained their use in adherence to the guidelines. While some of the non-adherence is associated with concerns about side effects, patient trust and the partnership with the doctor in agreeing preferences are major factors in treatment management (Hunot et al., 2007).[4]

Communication

Central to trust-building in healthcare is the communication of information to patients and their families. However, while the provision of information is a key determinant of patient and caregiver satisfaction, it is difficult to ascertain what the optimal level of information might be, by different individuals at different points in treatment and care. In a study of healthcare satisfaction for people with a first onset of psychosis, we noted the concerns and very low satisfaction of families for information-giving by psychiatric staff (Leavey et al., 1997). However, during the establishment of a family psycho-educational intervention based on information-giving, many families declared that they no longer needed healthcare information or they didn't wish to be reminded of the illness (Leavey et al., 2004).

Even further upstream, significant communication between agencies is deficient and that institutions and professions place boundaries between relationships. While such barriers can be partly explained by differences in disciplinary knowledge and terminology, they also arise from forms of professional protectionism. For example, while schoolteachers are generally more comfortable in addressing pupils' negative behaviours as disciplinary problems rather than expressions of emotional and psychological disorders, it is also the case that they are not trained to recognise and manage such problems and don't have the financial resources to do so. However, mental health services and schools tend to have minimal contact and information exchange about individual children and young people, even though this is likely to be mutually rewarding.

The protection of patient confidentiality is usually invoked as a reason for not sharing information, which in many cases may be sensible. However, in research on suicide and contact with services, there was a strong perception among families that they are excluded by healthcare professionals in providing important information that could have prevented deaths. In some cases, the information concerned concealed behaviours and discussions that were considered important to risk-assessment. Moreover, patients are commonly released from hospital into family care but information on the risk of suicide isn't provided to protect '*patient confidentiality*', despite the obvious challenges in their caring responsibilities. It is true that in some cases families may not provide protective environments, and information-sharing and involvement should be negligible, but most families offer a vital role in caring and support.

Collaborative care

Although the evidence suggests that collaborative care can have a significant impact on adherence, this requires additional resources and their costs will inevitably make the routinisation of collaboration unattractive to doctors or the healthcare providers (Vergouwen et al., 2003). However, it is often forgotten that most health care is provided by families and friends, without whom most healthcare systems would collapse. Thus, substantial evidence built over several decades, highlights the importance of family support for people living with mental illness – in providing material resources such as housing and food, but also maintaining the individual's life in the community, through encouraging medication adherence and routines of daily life. Importantly, they also provide love and human contact. However, the symptoms of schizophrenia or bi-polar disorder for example, are often challenging, and sometimes lead to a breakdown in management and care. Despite the obvious economic, social, and personal costs associated with family stress and relinquishment of care, there is a continuing lack of investment in family support interventions, across all diagnostic areas. Previously, I described how families become excluded as decision-making partners by clinical services, often with disastrous, sometime fatal, consequences. Too often, 'patient confidentiality' is interpreted too rigidly.

In a study of general practitioners' experiences of treating suicidal patients, a commonly reported concern was that family doctors feel out of their depth (Leavey et al., 2017). They readily acknowledged their limited confidence in this area. Because the risk factors for suicide are common but suicide as an event remains rare, when and how to intervene was a distressing predicament. 'Overreacting' to an individual's distress and summoning a psychiatrist risked patient mistrust and disengagement, while not reacting risked suicide. Prior to the restructuring of psychiatric services into a 'functional' split model in which psychiatrists are allocated to specialisms, the general practitioner could 'pick up a phone' to a familiar psychiatrist and discuss a patient's potential for suicide and activate advice and support. This valued model of collegial capital was replaced by an almost impenetrable impersonal structure of remote and disconnected managers. The aim, as is often the case, was to improve efficiency but the unintended consequence was to remove informal conduits of exchange that build interpersonal knowledge and trust into healthcare relationships which ultimately improve systems and patient care.

In Finland, the Open Dialogue Approach service for people experiencing mental health problems appears to show considerable promise in maintaining people in their own homes and communities by strengthening the individuals' support network. Thus, unlike traditional psychiatric services in the United Kingdom and the United States, family, friends, and sometimes colleagues, are meaningfully engaged in the care of the individual and supported in their understanding of the illness. The evidence thus far suggests that the Open Dialogue Approach as an integrative early-intervention system can produce improved health and social outcomes (Bergström et al., 2018). However, trust-building in psychiatric and other health services requires time and continuity of care, the maintenance of contact and knowledge with a clinician or group of clinicians is increasingly something of an ideal held by most patients, rather than a common experience within healthcare systems.

Notes

1 In terms of government and philanthropic funding, the provision for mental illness is low on the list of medical beneficiaries, even though almost 1 billion people worldwide currently experience a mental disorder costing US$1 trillion annually. Additionally, poor mental health overall, is estimated to cost the world economy approximately $2.5 trillion per year in poor health and reduced productivity in 2010, a cost projected to rise to $6 trillion by 2030 (Brohan et al., 2024).

2 In the United Kingdom, hundreds of individual hard-working and honest post-office workers were erroneously prosecuted for stealing money when all the time lurking in the computerised accounting system foisted upon all of them a digital malfunction was the real culprit. The infallibility of the computer was assumed rather than the honesty of the post office staff, many of whom were prosecuted and jailed; most lost their businesses, community respect and mental health. Several people took their own lives.

3 Importantly, there is much that we can do to build familiarity between young people and the medical profession through school-based interventions and adolescent-specific clinics.

4 Experience-Based Co-design (EBCD) is a potentially useful approach to understanding patients' needs and preferences for care in mental health services, adapted from its original use in cancer care and other health settings but the evidence thus far suggests major implementation challenges including problems in staff continuity and residual problems of asymmetry of power (Vennik et al., 2016).

References

Bateman, A., Brown, D., & Pedder, J. (2000). *Introduction to psychotherapy: An outline of psychodynamic principles and practice*. Routledge.

Bergström, T., Seikkula, J., Alakare, B., Mäki, P., Köngäs-Saviaro, P., Taskila, J. J., Tolvanen, A., & Aaltonen, J. (2018). The family-oriented open dialogue approach in the treatment of first-episode psychosis: Nineteen-year outcomes. *Psychiatry Research, 270,* 168–175. https://doi.org/10.1016/j.psychres.2018.09.039

Brohan, E., Chowdhary, N., Dua, T., Barbui, C., Thornicroft, G., Kestel, D., Ali, A., Assanangkornchai, S., Brodaty, H., Carli, V., El Chammay, R., Chang, O., Collins, P. Y., Cuijpers, P., Dowrick, C., Eaton, J., Ferri, C. P., Fortes, S., Hengartner, M. P., ... Sumi, Y. (2024). The WHO mental health gap action programme for mental, neurological, and substance use conditions: The new and updated guideline recommendations. *The Lancet Psychiatry.* https://doi.org/10.1016/S2215-0366(23)00370-X

Carel, H., & Kidd, I. J. (2014). Epistemic injustice in healthcare: A philosophical analysis. *Medicine, Health Care and Philosophy, 17*(4), 529–540. https://doi.org/10.1007/s11019-014-9560-2

Cook, K. S., Kramer, R. M., Thom, D. H., Stepanikova, I., Mollborn, S. B., & Cooper, R. M. (2004). Trust and distrust in patient-physician relationships: Perceived determinants of high- and low-trust relationships in managed care settings In M. Kramer & K. Cook (Eds.), *Trust and distrust in organizations: Dilemmas and approaches.* Russell Sage.

Gratzer, D., & Goldbloom, D. (2019). Open for business: Chatbots, e-therapies, and the future of psychiatry. *The Canadian Journal of Psychiatry, 64*(7), 453–455. https://doi.org/10.1177/0706743719850057

Hunot, V. M., Horne, R., Leese, M. N., & Churchill, R. C. (2007). A cohort study of adherence to antidepressants in primary care: The influence of antidepressant concerns and treatment preferences. *Primary Care Companion to the Journal Clinical Psychiatry, 9*(2), 91–99. https://doi.org/10.4088/pcc.v09n0202

Kleinman, A. (1988). *The illness narratives: Suffering, healing, and the human condition.* Basic Books.

Leavey, G., Gulamhussein, S., Papadopoulos, C., Johnson-Sabine, E., Blizard, B., & King, M. (2004). A randomised controlled intervention for families of patients with a first onset of psychosis. *Psychological Medicine, 34,* 423–431.

Leavey, G., King, M., Cole, E., Hoar, A., & Sabine, E. (1997). First onset psychotic illness; patients' and relatives' satisfaction with services. *British Journal of Psychiatry, 170,* 53–57.

Leavey, G., Mallon, S., Rondon-Sulbaran, J., Galway, K., Rosato, M., & Hughes, L. (2017). The failure of suicide prevention in primary care: Family and GP perspectives - a qualitative study. *BMC Psychiatry, 17*(1), 369. https://doi.org/10.1186/s12888-017-1508-7

Metzl, J. M., & Hansen, H. (2018). Structural competency and psychiatry. *JAMA Psychiatry, 75*(2), 115–116. https://doi.org/10.1001/jamapsychiatry.2017.3891

Monteith, S., Glenn, T., Geddes, J. R., Whybrow, P. C., Achtyes, E., & Bauer, M. (2024). Artificial intelligence and increasing misinformation. *The British Journal of Psychiatry, 224*(2), 33–35. https://doi.org/10.1192/bjp.2023.136

Sakakibara, E. (2023). Epistemic injustice in the therapeutic relationship in psychiatry. *Theoretical Medicine and Bioethics, 44*(5), 477–502. https://doi.org/10.1007/s11017-023-09627-1

Vennik, F. D., Van de Bovenkamp, H. M., Putters, K., & Grit, K. J. (2016). Co-production in healthcare: Rhetoric and practice. *International Review of Administrative Sciences, 82*(1), 150–168.

Vergouwen, A. C., Bakker, A., Katon, W. J., Verheij, T. J., & Koerselman, F. (2003). Improving adherence to antidepressants: A systematic review of interventions. *Journal of Clinical Psychiatry, 64*(12), 1415–1420. https://doi.org/10.4088/jcp.v64n1203

Index

Printed in the United States
by Baker & Taylor Publisher Services